T0224709

Understanding Inferential Statistics

Markus Janczyk • Roland Pfister

Understanding Inferential Statistics

From A for Significance Test to Z
for Confidence Interval

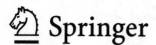 Springer

Markus Janczyk
Research Methods and Cognitive Psychology
University of Bremen
Bremen, Germany

Roland Pfister
General Psychology
Trier University
Trier, Germany

ISBN 978-3-662-66785-9   ISBN 978-3-662-66786-6   (eBook)
https://doi.org/10.1007/978-3-662-66786-6

The first draft of the translation was compiled with the help of artificial intelligence (machine translation by the service DeepL.com). The authors subsequently revised this draft thoroughly in terms of content and style.

This Springer imprint is published by the registered company Springer-Verlag GmbH, DE, part of Springer Nature.
The registered company address is: Heidelberger Platz 3, 14197 Berlin, Germany

Paper in this product is recyclable.

Preface to the English Translation (3rd Edition)

This book originated from a joint endeavor of the authors to provide two things: a concise introduction to the basic mechanics of statistical inference combined with hands-on guidance on how to put these mechanics into action. Owing to the native language of the authors, the book was initially published in German, and we are happy to present this translation of the book's 3rd edition. We had wanted to translate this work ever since the original book saw the light of day in 2013 but shied away from putting this ambitious plan into action at first. Matters changed when the team at Springer approached us in April 2021, kindly offering an AI-powered translation.

The following text is based on what this AI had crafted. When browsing through the text, however, we couldn't help but feel that some parts of the text had an interesting lyrical quality—including headlines such as "For deepening", "A small anticipation for later", or concepts such as sampling "with putting back" (citing from the original draft). Other parts felt overly close to the original phrasing so that the English text did not come across particularly naturally. Idioms also proved to be a challenge for the AI, rendering some parts difficult to understand. We, therefore, rolled up our sleeves and started revising the original draft from the ground up.

The final prose thus is an eclectic mix of machine grammar blended in with attempts to distill our German formulations into readable English. Despite our best efforts, there will likely be paragraphs that we did not revise sufficiently strongly. The book's subtitle "From A for Significance Test to Z for Confidence Interval" may come to mind, though we are happy to confirm that this subtitle has also bewildered the readership of the German edition (and we are still very happy with it). Other paragraphs may have been changed for the worse by our well-intentioned attempts. While revising the text, we came across some additional errors that were still present in the German 3rd edition. These have been corrected of course. In addition, we have slightly adapted the references to include more English-language literature (the translated online material is available at https://doi.org/10.1007/978-3-662-66786-6_1. Our hope is that the overall text manages to reach its goal of showcasing how inferential statistics work and how to apply these procedures competently and efficiently. We would be thrilled to get feedback on whether this is indeed the case.

Bremen, Germany   Markus Janczyk
Würzburg, Germany   Roland Pfister
August 2022

Preface to the 3rd Edition

The 4 years since the publication of the 2nd edition have seen extensive discussions about statistical methods in various disciplines. The most prominent discussion relates to increasingly frequent calls to replace classical inferential statistical methods with alternative concepts, as discussed for instance by the American Statistical Association in a recently published issue (Wasserstein et al. 2019). A common criticism here is that inferential statistical measures are often misinterpreted and misunderstood (Hubbard 2011).

We are convinced that such claims go a little too far. Rather, we believe, classical methods such as null hypothesis significance testing are a valid and useful method of data analysis—provided they are used correctly. Correctly using these tools, however, requires a solid understanding of the logic underlying classical inferential statistical methods. This was and is the primary aim of this book. At the same time, in light of the current discussion, we consider it useful to look at other methods of statistical inference as well. In addition to the previous discussion of confidence intervals and effect sizes (which are sometimes referred to as "new statistics"), we have thus expanded the 3rd edition with a new chapter on Bayesian alternatives. As with the presentation of the classical methods, this chapter focuses on the logic of the corresponding methods, followed by a separate description of how to implement them with hands-on examples. We hope that this description enables an informed assessment of the available statistical toolbox by revealing the advantages and disadvantages of both approaches.

The addition of Bayesian methods is of course not the only change in the 3rd edition. Rather, we have expanded on the introductory sections that derive the logic behind classical inferential statistics so that these sections are now more comprehensive, and we hope: also (even) more intuitive. To this end, we consistently present data examples and simulations based on clearly defined populations to give a feel for how inferential statistical analyses work. Of course, we have also made other minor changes and optimizations (and also revised the online material; see www.springer.com/978-3-662-59908-2). We hope that this book will continue to provide a useful resource for students, teachers, and researchers.

Bremen, Germany   Markus Janczyk
Würzburg, Germany   Roland Pfister
August 2019

Preface to the 2nd Edition

The first edition of this book has now been available for about 2 years. We are pleased that the book and its concept have been welcomed by the scientific community, and we are glad to present the second edition. We thank all readers of the previous edition, particularly for all comments, suggestions, and constructive feedback.

The basic approach and most of the content has stayed the same as in the first edition: Our aim still is to give a simple and comprehensible approach to what we consider the most important and common methods of inferential statistics, without getting bogged down in details. There are occasional additions, however, in which we address current issues and controversies that we consider relevant for the future development of the field. In addition, we have corrected minor errors and made linguistic revisions in many sections. We have also extended the online material (see the URL in the preface to the 1st edition), in particular by adding examples for SPSS syntax for all analyses. We hope that the book will continue to be received well and we are looking forward to receiving new comments and suggestions.

Tübingen, Germany   Markus Janczyk
Würzburg, Germany   Roland Pfister
October 2015

Preface to the 1st Edition

Empirical studies are the cornerstone of scientific progress in many disciplines across the natural and social sciences. Psychology, sociology, educational science, or neuroscience require solid knowledge about how to obtain and evaluate data. Correctly interpreting the results of an empirical study therefore is a central skill in these fields, and acquiring this skill is a key part of academic education. This book is primarily aimed at students of these fields, but also at advanced researchers working and teaching in these fields.

The aim of this book is to provide a graspable approach to common procedures in inferential statistics, enabling its readers to apply such procedures competently in their own work. We have paid particular attention to the basic logic of inferential statistical procedures, with the intention of providing a thorough understanding and emphasizing connections between different procedures. These theoretical aspects are complemented by hands-on examples on how to apply each procedure with SPSS and R, as well as examples for how to present corresponding results.

Reading this book requires basic knowledge of descriptive statistics, as summarized in the first chapter. The three following chapters are devoted to the theoretical foundation of inferential statistics, providing the necessary tools for understanding any type of inferential statistical test. The remaining chapters then cover the most important procedures, from t-tests to analyses of variance, concluding with correlation and regression analyses. Important contemporary topics are covered as well, including confidence intervals, effect sizes, and the power of significance tests.

We have tried to avoid unnecessary formulas and details in the main text of the book, thus allowing for occasional mathematical vagueness. For readers who are particularly interested in such detail, however, we have included sections with grey backgrounds in the text; these contain formal notes and derivations, background knowledge, and other information to support the main text. Supplementary documents, as well as exemplary data sets and annotated analysis scripts can also be found as online material at http://www.springer.com/de/book/9783662471050 [in German]. The figures and illustrations of this book are also available at this link for use as course material. Although this book is written in German [and now in English as well, as of the 3rd edition], we have used decimal-point notation (instead of the German decimal comma) as commonly found in scientific publications and widely used by many statistical programs. Furthermore, where we present examples on how to report statistical results, we have followed the guidelines of the American Psychological Association.

We would like to thank all people without whom this book would have appeared earlier than it did, but certainly also in a much less comprehensible and accurate state. These are first and foremost Katharina Schwarz, Thomas Göb, and Stefan Friedrich, whose careful review revealed quite a few inconsistencies and expositional issues, thus playing a key role in shaping the final version of this book. Thank you also to numerous students who vetted individual chapters for their comprehensibility. This book would probably not have been published at all without the mediating interventions of Alexander "Take your time" Heinemann, who mediated many heated discussions between the two authors. Wilfried Kunde granted us the necessary resources and the best possible working conditions at his chair for realizing this project. We are also thankful for the great support by the staff of Springer who supervised this project: Alice Blanck, Agnes Herrmann, Clemens Heine, and Niels Peter Thomas. Finally, we would like to thank Dieter Heyer (Halle), Gisela Müller-Plath (Berlin), and Rainer Scheuchenpflug (Würzburg) for their contagious enthusiasm for statistics and research methods.

Bremen, Germany   Markus Janczyk
Würzburg, Germany   Roland Pfister
November 2012

Contents

Introduction and Descriptive Statistics

1

Progress in many scientific disciplines builds on creative ideas and questions that can only be answered on the basis of empirical data. Similarly, predictions from theories can only be tested using empirical data. In this context, scientific work often claims to uncover universally valid regularities about causal mechanisms or relationships between different variables. This goal of deriving general claims from observable data is surprisingly challenging: Whereas the (specific) question of whether the sun is shining right now can be answered by looking out of the window, there is no way to provide a direct answer to the following questions—taken from the field of psychological research:

- Is lying cognitively more challenging than responding truthfully?
- Do socially anxious and non-socially anxious individuals differ in their gaze behavior?
- Is memory performance better for events that conform to a schema or for atypical events?
- Does employee satisfaction differ between teams with participative versus authoritarian leadership?

Answering such questions requires the methods of inferential statistics. We will provide a brief introduction to the basic logic of this approach in the following section.

Inferential statistics require a correct description of existing data. The methods of **descriptive statistics** (Sect. 1.3) fulfill precisely this role. They allow expressing essential aspects of a data set in simple and clear terms. However, they can only be used to make statements about this existing data set, for example, about the mean of a measured variable.

Supplementary Information The online version contains supplementary material available at (https://doi.org/10.1007/978-3-662-66786-6_1).

Any statement that goes beyond these directly observed measures requires the methods of inferential statistics.

1.1   Why Inferential Statistics?

The exemplary questions from the field of psychology raised in the beginning intentionally imply general statements; they should apply to people in general—perhaps not to the same degree for each individual person, but at least on average. Moreover, this claim often includes a temporal dimension, so that it explicitly includes people who have lived before or will live in the future. It is therefore obvious that the set of potential cases—the so-called population—cannot be fully investigated. This is why empirical disciplines work with so-called **samples** that are drawn from the **population**, and we will come back to this procedure in the following chapters.

The use of samples from a population raises the question as to how measures from such samples can be used to assess the validity of generalized claims. In other words: Which observations can we reasonably expect to generalize beyond the available sample?

Central to the understanding of this process is the concept of variability. In this regard, inferential statistics distinguishes between (at least) two types of variability: systematic variability, which is due to the mechanism or correlation under study, and random variability, which derives from an unknown source or a source not currently of interest to an investigation. As an example of these two types of variability, we would like to follow up on the last psychological question raised at the beginning ("Does employee satisfaction differ between teams with participative versus authoritarian leadership?"). If we now surveyed a number of employees from both types of teams regarding their satisfaction, the answers across both samples will differ depending on each employee's personal experiences, expectations, and attitudes. By comparing the mean satisfaction of the employees of both types of teams, one obtains an estimate of the systematic variability, that is, the difference in satisfaction that derives from team membership. The question now is whether this difference in mean satisfaction between the two types of teams (the systematic variability) is substantially larger than the to-be-expected variability of the individual measures around the corresponding mean value (the random variability). Intuitively, we can speak of a statistically "significant" difference if the systematic variability is large and the random variability is relatively small.

It is less obvious to determine what exact difference between systematic and random variability qualifies as sufficiently large. Precisely this is the question that inferential statistics aims to specify and formalize to provide explicit decision rules as to which conclusions are appropriate based on which data.

Already this simplified description of the agenda of inferential statistics implies that inferential statements are always statements about probabilities. Decisions based on (estimated) probabilities can never claim to be an ultimate proof. Rather, inferential statistical results necessarily come with the possibility of a decision error.

Correctly applying and interpreting inferential statistical methods thus requires a sound understanding of the underlying decision process and relevant sources of error. We will cover these aspects in detail in the chapters of this book.

In Depth 1.1: History
Inferential statistics are ubiquitous in contemporary research, and they form the backbone of many scientific disciplines. Nevertheless, the use of such methods for data analysis is a surprisingly recent development in the history of science that has started only about 100 years ago (e.g., Fienberg 1992).

The form of inferential statistics mainly considered in this book is called "classical inferential statistics" or "null hypothesis significance testing." It is probably the most widely used statistical method, particularly in the psychological literature. Nevertheless, there are also several alternative approaches, of which Bayesian statistics in particular have attracted increasing attention in recent years (see Chap. 12). We will comment on the state of this current discussion at various points.

1.2 Important Mathematical Notations

1.2.1 The Summation Sign

The summation sign plays an important role in this book (and also in statistics in general) and is used as an abbreviated notation for a sum. As an example, consider the data from five studied cases—for example, people—on a variable X. In the following, we will denote variables in uppercase letters whereas individual, concrete values on these variables come as lowercase letters:

$$x_1 = 3, \qquad x_2 = 5, \qquad x_3 = 1, \qquad x_4 = 0, \qquad x_5 = -1.$$

Figure 1.1 summarizes the components of the **summation sign**. Following this notation, we can write the sum $x_1 + x_2 + x_3 + x_4 + x_5 = 8$ as:

$$\sum_{i=1}^{5} x_i = 8.$$

The summation sign is especially relevant when considering not only five but an infinite number of values, or situations for which we cannot know the exact number of values; these situations are commonplace in statistics. In Formula 1.1 we consider n values, without further specifying the exact number n. This is the case, for example, when the

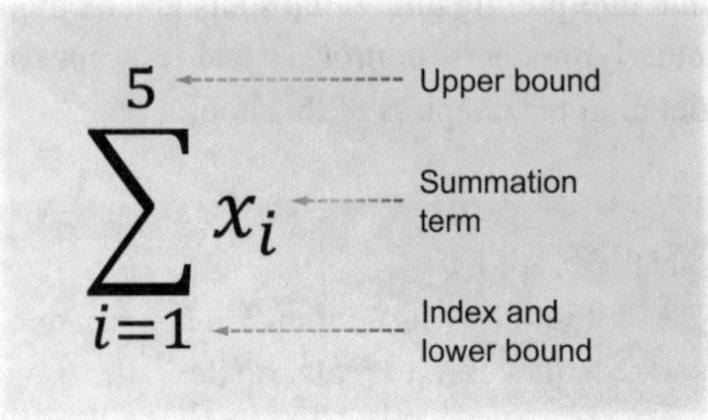

$$\sum_{i=1}^{5} x_i$$

- 5 — Upper bound
- x_i — Summation term
- $i=1$ — Index and lower bound

Fig. 1.1 The summation sign and its components. Here, i denotes the *index of summation*, though any letter may be used as an index. The number 1 is the *lower bound*, 5 is the *upper bound* of the index, and the expression after the summation sign (in this case x_i) represents the *summation term*, i.e., the elements to be summed up

sample size is not (yet) known and formulas should therefore be kept general to apply to any sample size:

$$x_1 + x_2 + \ldots + x_{n-1} + x_n = \sum_{i=1}^{n} x_i. \tag{1.1}$$

Some *important calculation rules with the summation sign* are:

- Let a be a constant real number (shorthand notation: $a \in \mathbb{R}$), then:

$$\sum_{i=1}^{n} a x_i = a \sum_{i=1}^{n} x_i.$$

- Let $a \in \mathbb{R}$, then:

$$\sum_{i=1}^{n} a = \underbrace{a + a + a + \ldots + a}_{n \text{ times}} = na.$$

- Let X and Y be two variables, then:

$$\sum_{i=1}^{n} (x_i + y_i) = \sum_{i=1}^{n} x_i + \sum_{i=1}^{n} y_i.$$

- A similar equation is *not* generally true for multiplication:

$$\sum_{i=1}^{n}(x_i \cdot y_i) \neq \sum_{i=1}^{n} x_i \cdot \sum_{i=1}^{n} y_i.$$

- A frequent source of error is also the position of the exponent:

$$\sum_{i=1}^{n} x_i^2 \neq \left(\sum_{i=1}^{n} x_i\right)^2.$$

Considering the five values of the example, the results are

$$\sum_{i=1}^{5}(x_i^2) = 36 \quad \text{and} \quad \left(\sum_{i=1}^{5} x_i\right)^2 = 64.$$

1.2.2   Set Theory and its Notations

In this section we give a brief overview of notations from set theory that we will use in the following.

Sets consist of a "collection of elements". Sets are usually denoted by uppercase letters and their elements by lowercase letters. If, for example, a is an **element of the set** A, this is expressed by $a \in A$. The set of the natural numbers is denoted by $\mathbb{N}$ and the set of real numbers by $\mathbb{R}$. If certain sets are introduced explicitly, their elements are written in curly brackets. For the set A of the numbers 1, 2, 3, and 4, we can write:

$$A = \{1, 2, 3, 4\} \quad \text{or} \quad A = \{1, \ldots, 4\} \quad \text{or} \quad A = \{x \,|\, x \in \mathbb{N} \text{ and } 1 \leq x \leq 4\}.$$

All three variants denote the same set; the third variant reads "A is the set of all numbers x for which holds: x is an element of the natural numbers and lies between 1 and 4 (both inclusive)".

Occasionally we will use set notation in connection with the summation sign. If we wanted to sum up all elements of the set A, this sum can be written as:

$$\sum_{a \in A} a = 10.$$

In addition, we will sometimes perform a particular calculation for different groups or conditions. This can be expressed by the so-called "alloquantor" $\forall$. The character $\forall$ is read as "for all". As an example, let us consider three values x_1, x_2, and x_3 to each of which we want to add 10. This can be written as:

$$x_i' = x_i + 10 \qquad \forall i \in \{1, 2, 3\}.$$

1.2.3 Variable Transformations

Sometimes we will create a new variable from an existing one by multiplying the values with a certain factor and/or adding certain values to them. If, for example, we wanted to create a new variable $aX + b$ from the variable X, this would mean the following: We take each value x_i, multiply it with a, and then add b to the result. This procedure is called a **linear transformation**.

Similarly, we can generate new variables by combining two existing variables, for example, by adding or multiplying them. If, for example, there are two variables X and Y, then the new variable $Z = X + Y$ denotes the addition of the corresponding pairs of measured values: $z_i = x_i + y_i$.

1.3 Descriptive Statistics

The first step in any analysis of empirical data is describing the data at hand; this is the field of descriptive statistics. Two particularly important measures here are the *arithmetic mean* and the *(sample) variance*. To illustrate these measures, we consider two exemplary data sets as given in Table 1.1. The following calculations refer to these two samples.

1.3.1 Arithmetic Mean

To calculate the **arithmetic mean** $\bar{X}$ ("mean value"),[1] all individual measured values are first added up and the sum is then divided by the number n of measured values. Using the

Table 1.1 Two exemplary data sets of $n = 12$ participants each. Each participant contributes one measured value to the variables X_1 and X_2

	Participant											
	1	2	3	4	5	6	7	8	9	10	11	12
Example 1 (X_1)	4	4	4	4	5	5	5	5	6	6	6	6
Example 2 (X_2)	5	5	5	5	6	6	6	4	4	4	3	7

---

[1] There are different notations for the arithmetic mean; we use $\bar{X}$ and M_X interchangeably.

summation sign, this procedure can be written for the n measured values $x_1, x_2, \ldots, x_n$ as:

$$\bar{X} = M_X = \frac{1}{n} \sum_{i=1}^{n} x_i = \frac{\sum_{i=1}^{n} x_i}{n}. \tag{1.2}$$

If we apply this formula to Example 1 from Table 1.1, the resulting mean is

$$\bar{X}_1 = M_{X_1} = \frac{4+4+4+4+5+5+5+5+6+6+6+6}{12} = \frac{60}{12} = 5.$$

The same applies to Example 2: $\bar{X}_2 = M_{X_2} = 5$. Some *important properties of the arithmetic mean* are:

- If we calculate the mean of n values and then compute the difference of each measured value x_i to the mean value $\bar{X}$ and add up these differences, the result is always zero:

$$\sum_{i=1}^{n} (x_i - \bar{X}) = 0.$$

- The mean of a linear transformation $aX + b$ corresponds to the linear transformation of the mean of the original variable. Thus, let $a, b \in \mathbb{R}$, then:

$$M_{aX+b} = a M_X + b.$$

- The following relation holds for the addition of two variables X and Y:

$$M_{X+Y} = M_X + M_Y.$$

- The same is *not* generally true for multiplication:

$$M_{X \cdot Y} \neq M_X \cdot M_Y.$$

1.3.2 Sample Variance

As we have seen, the mean values of both variables in Table 1.1 are identical. However, if we visualize the example data with a histogram (Fig. 1.2), the two variables still appear to be quite different. This is evident in the ranges of values as well as in the different shapes of the histograms. These and other properties can be captured by *measures of variability*. We consider three such measures that are important here: the sample variance, the standard deviation, and the standard error (of the mean). These measures reveal properties of the data that cannot be captured by the mean and are therefore needed to fully describe the data.

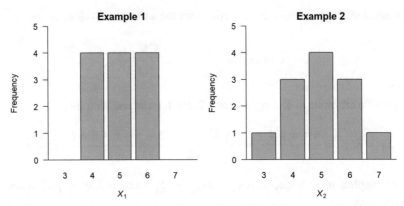

Fig. 1.2 Histograms of the two exemplary data sets from Table 1.1

The **variance** S_X^2 is the mean squared deviation of the measured values from their mean. If $\bar{X}$ is the mean of n measured values $x_1, x_2, \ldots, x_n$, then their variance is:

$$S_X^2 = \frac{\sum_{i=1}^n (x_i - \bar{X})^2}{n}. \tag{1.3}$$

The deviations of the individual measured values x_i from the mean $\bar{X}$ are thus squared and summed up. Finally, this sum is divided by n.[2] Squaring prevents the sum of the deviations from always being zero. If it is still zero, then all values x_i of the variable X are identical as is their mean:

$$S_X^2 \geq 0 \quad \text{and} \quad S_X^2 = 0 \Leftrightarrow x_1 = x_2 = \ldots = x_n = \bar{X}.$$

The variance of the data from Example 1 is calculated as follows:

$$S_{X_1}^2 = \frac{(4-5)^2 + (4-5)^2 + (4-5)^2 + (4-5)^2}{12}$$

$$+ \frac{(5-5)^2 + (5-5)^2 + (5-5)^2 + (5-5)^2}{12}$$

$$+ \frac{(6-5)^2 + (6-5)^2 + (6-5)^2 + (6-5)^2}{12} = \frac{8}{12} = 0.667.$$

---

[2] Some textbooks define the variance slightly differently and divide not by n, but by $n-1$. When computing descriptive statistics of a sample, however, we should use the version introduced here; in Sect. 3.4 we will clarify this difference.

If we calculate the variance for Example 2, we see that the apparent differences between both samples are actually reflected in a different value:

$$S_{X_2}^2 = \frac{(5-5)^2 + (5-5)^2 + \ldots + (3-5)^2 + (7-5)^2}{12} = \frac{14}{12} = 1.167.$$

The variance S_X^2 is also the starting point for two other important measures of descriptive statistics. The **standard deviation** S_X is the square root of the variance:

$$S_X = \sqrt{S_X^2}. \tag{1.4}$$

Finally, to calculate the **standard error of the mean** SE_M, the standard deviation is divided by the square root of the sample size n:

$$SE_M = \frac{S_X}{\sqrt{n}}. \tag{1.5}$$

1.4   Statistical Software: R and SPSS

There are numerous commercial and non-commercial programs available for computing statistical tests. Here we introduce examples of two of the most common software packages: R as a widespread non-commercial program and SPSS as a widely used commercial package. The eventual choice between these and other computer programs is a subjective one, without a clear right or wrong answer. To facilitate this choice, and to showcase the flavor of both programs we will compute the measures discussed so far with both programs.

In some of the following chapters we will calculate concrete examples with both programs. More often than not, these procedures are only one of many possible solutions within each program.

1.4.1   Statistical Computing with R

There are numerous introductions available for the statistical package R (www.r-project. org), both on the internet (e.g., on the stated homepage) and in printed form (e.g., deVries and Meys 2012; Ligges 2009; Wollschläger 2010). At the same time, R offers extensive possibilities for statistical analyses and visualization of data, so that giving this program a try is certainly worthwhile. Working with R is especially smooth when using additional programs to interface the R language. One such interface is RStudio (www.rstudio.org).

Here we will revisit the exemplary calculations for Example 1 in R by first creating the variable X_1:

```
X1 <- c(4, 4, 4, 4, 5, 5, 5, 5, 6, 6, 6, 6)
```

The mean of this variable can be calculated easily with the R function `mean()`, and we get the corresponding output directly:

```
mean(X1)

5
```

To calculate the variance of X_1 we convert Formula 1.3 into R:

```
variance <- (1/length(X1))*sum((X1-mean(X1))^2)
variance

0.6666667
```

The standard deviation is calculated as the square root of this result:

```
sqrt(variance)

0.8164966
```

Of course, R also has functions to calculate the variance and standard deviation directly, namely `var(X1)` and `sd(X1)`—but these give different results than the calculation by hand. This is due to R not calculating the sample variance, but the estimator for the so-called population variance—a difference we will explain in Sect. 3.4.

The examples in later chapters will use larger data sets. These data are often available as tables, but they are also provided in electronic form in the online material for this book. All files for R are located in the eponymous folder; data files come with the file extension `.dat`, commented syntax files are `.R` files. To be able to read existing data into R, we first use `setwd()` to set the path to the directory in which the file is located. Then we use the `read.table()` command to read the data and assign it to a data frame named `data`:

```
setwd("C:/understanding_inferential_statistics/R/")
data <- read.table("1_exemplary_data.dat",
                header = TRUE, sep = "\t")
```

The option `header = TRUE` means that the first line of the file contains the variable names, and `sep = "\t"` means that the individual variables and their values are separated by tab stops.

It is also possible to access the variables of the resulting data frame (X1 and X2) individually. This is done either by column index

```
data[1]    # access only the variable in column 1 (X1)
```

or via the so-called "naming" function:

```
data$X1   # access only the variable named X1
```

If we want to make the variables of the data frame directly available, we can load the content of the data frame data with the attach() function (see the online material for details):

```
X1    # >> error message
attach(data)
X1    # displays the variable X1
```

The functionality of the R base software can also be extended by installing add-on packages. The most important package for our purposes is named ez (Lawrence 2016) and provides a number of useful features, including evaluation and display of factorial designs; we will return to these features in later chapters. Other additional features are provided by the package schoRsch, which was created by the authors of this book and provides easy and quick access to the output of various statistical tests, among other things (Pfister and Janczyk 2016). We will also refer to this package in the following chapters. We therefore recommend installing at least these two packages.

1.4.2   The Statistical Package SPSS

SPSS is a classic commercial statistical package and is still widely used. SPSS is shorthand for *Statistical Package for the Social Sciences* and is the original and current name of the software; the program was also distributed under the name PASW for a short time. The examples and screenshots in this book were created with program version 27 throughout.

We assume a basic understanding of the program, for which numerous introductions exist on the internet. A comprehensive description of the program can also be found in McCormick et al. (2015) or Janssen and Laatz (2010). In addition to the graphical user interface, SPSS also offers the possibility of using syntax, and we highly recommend using this latter option after getting used to the workflow of SPSS. In this book, we mainly describe the graphical user interface (which can generate syntax using the "Paste" button); corresponding examples of pure syntax files are available in the online material. The online material also contains the data files (.sav) for the examples used later. In order to understand the structure of syntax files, it can sometimes be helpful to consult the *Command Syntax Reference*, which can be accessed via the menu item *Help*.

Descriptive Statistics

	N	Mean	Std. Deviation	Variance
X1	12	5.00	.853	.727
X2	12	5.00	1.128	1.273
Valid N (listwise)	12			

Fig. 1.3 SPSS output of common descriptive statistics

As an exercise, we will compute descriptive statistics for the two example variables. To do this, we open the file 1_exemplary_data.sav and then select the menu

Analyze > Descriptive Statistics > Descriptives...

Under *Options* we check the boxes for *Mean, Standard Deviation*, and *Variance* and confirm with *OK*.[3] This generates an output table as shown in Fig. 1.3. The mean values obviously agree with the values calculated by hand whereas the variances differ from our manual results. This difference is due to the fact that SPSS (just like R) does not calculate the sample variance, but an estimator for the population variance—a difference that we will discuss in detail in Sect. 3.4 (manually calculating the sample variance, as described above for R, cannot be done easily in SPSS).

---

[3] Clicking *Paste* instead of *OK* will convert the requested operation to syntax that can be saved and re-run later on.

Introduction to Inferential Statistics 1: Random Variables

2

The previous chapter focused on describing concrete samples with the methods of descriptive statistics, that is, it focused on situations where we know the values of each element of the sample and we can therefore compute various measures from them, for example, the arithmetic mean and the variance of the measured values. We will now try to derive statements about the underlying population from a sample. This is the task of **inferential statistics**. Before we turn to the important distinction between sample and population in Chap. 3, we introduce some additional mathematical concepts here. In this context, we consider what values a variable *could* have in theory. To do this, we draw on concepts such as *random experiments* and *random variables and their distributions*. We will introduce these concepts using the more intuitive case of discrete random variables and then apply the concepts to the case of continuous random variables.

2.1 Discrete Random Variables

2.1.1 The Concept of Random Variables

Many processes can be repeated an arbitrary number of times under constant conditions, and yet their outcome is random. Such processes are called **random experiments**. A typical example is tossing a coin: There are two possible outcomes, head and tail, and the actual outcome occurs by chance. The set of all possible outcomes is usually referred to as Ω (an uppercase Omega), its elements as ω (a lowercase omega). Hence, in the coin example $\Omega = \{\text{head, tail}\}$. Another example is randomly drawing a card from a card deck. In the following examples, we use the 32 cards of a standard set of Skat cards—a traditional game in German-speaking countries (https://en.wikipedia.org/wiki/Skat_(card_game)). The following considerations build on this example and are illustrated in Fig. 2.1

© Springer-Verlag GmbH Germany, part of Springer Nature 2023
M. Janczyk, R. Pfister, *Understanding Inferential Statistics*,
https://doi.org/10.1007/978-3-662-66786-6_2

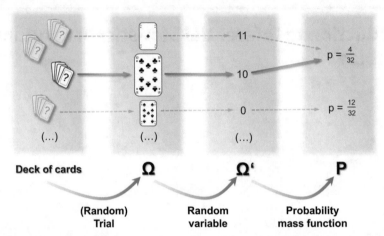

Fig. 2.1 Illustration of a (discrete) random variable and its probability mass function based on the example of drawing a card from a deck of 32 Skat cards. The random experiment can be repeated for any number of times (in theory) as indicated by the gray card decks and corresponding dashed arrows. Each iteration is called a trial and will result in its own, random card value

When drawing a card at random from such a deck, there are 32 different outcomes of this random experiment including, for example, Queen of Hearts, Jack of Spades, Ten of Clubs, etc.—the set Ω has 32 different elements. Now we are usually not interested in the card "itself" (i.e., the physical object), but we are interested in one of its properties. In addition to its symbol, the Skat player is particularly interested in the card's value.[1] Figure 2.1, for instance, shows the Ten of Clubs and this card has the value 10. We capture the card's characteristic of interest in a second set Ω' ("Omega prime"). In other words, each element of Ω, that is: each possible outcome of the random experiment, is assigned a (real) number. This is the purpose of so-called **random variables**. We could now repeat the random experiment as often as we like; its outcome, and thus the resulting card value, can differ across trials.

Similarly, randomly drawing a person (or more generally: a unit of investigation) from a set of persons can be regarded as a random experiment. Since every person of this set can be the outcome of the random experiment, this set of persons defines the set of all possible outcomes, that is, Ω. In this case, too, we are often not interested in the person "per se", but in certain values that represent an attribute of this person, for example, their age, height, IQ, score on a certain personality test, etc. In mathematical terms, this measurement boils down to assigning a real number (e.g., the person's height in cm) to an element of the set Ω—thus a random variable.

---

[1] Skat rules define the following values: Seven, Eight, and Nine = 0, Jack = 2, Queen = 3, King = 4, Ten = 10, and Ace = 11.

We denote random variables with bold Latin uppercase letters, for example, X, and they usually consist of two sets: The first set of all possible outcomes is Ω and the second set Ω'. The latter is usually a subset of $\mathbb{R}$. A random variable further assigns to each $\omega \in \Omega$ an element (i.e., a number) of Ω'. We speak of a **discrete random variable**, whenever Ω' has a finite number of elements (as in the card-drawing example or also when, e.g., measuring the gender of a person). If Ω' has an infinite number of elements, we speak of a continuous random variable (e.g., when measuring the height of a person, which could theoretically take any of an infinite number of different values if we only measured precisely enough). In the example of drawing a card in a game of Skat we have $\Omega' = \{0, 2, 3, 4, 10, 11\}$. Each realization of the random experiment "drawing one card at random" is thus assigned one of the card values 0, 2, 3, 4, 10, or 11.

In Depth 2.1: Formal Definition of Random Variables

Formally, a random variable is defined as follows: Let Ω be a set of possible outcomes of a random experiment and let Ω' be another (non-empty) set. A random variable X assigns to each $\omega \in \Omega$ an element of Ω'. It is therefore a mapping from Ω to Ω':

$$X : \Omega \to \Omega'.$$

Often Ω' is a subset of $\mathbb{R} : \Omega' \subseteq \mathbb{R}$.

In probability theory, the outcome of a random experiment is also called the result and the set Ω is also called the **sample space**. The term "result" should not be confused with the colloquial usage in the sense of "result of a study".

2.1.2 Probability Mass Functions

Building on the above steps, we are now interested in the probability of observing a certain value from Ω' as the result of a single trial of the random experiment. For this, we need the so-called **probability mass function** of the random variable and, as an example, we consider again the deck of Skat cards. Four of the 32 cards are aces, and these are the only cards that have a value of 11. The probability of obtaining a card value of 11 when drawing a single card from the full deck is thus $p_{11} = \frac{4}{32}$. The probability of obtaining a card value of 0 with a single draw is higher, because a total of 12 cards come with this value, that is, $p_0 = \frac{12}{32}$. Figure 2.2 illustrates this probability mass function.

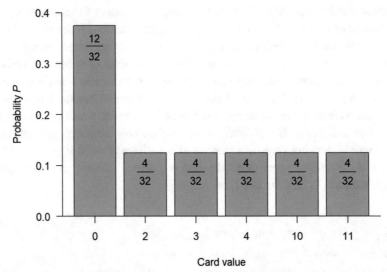

Fig. 2.2 Probability mass function of a discrete random variable. The underlying random experiment again assumes that we draw a single card from a full Skat deck of 32 cards and assess the resulting card value

---

In Depth 2.2: Formal Definition of Probability Mass Functions

Formally, a probability mass function f is a mapping that assigns a number to each element from Ω', namely its probability of occurrence. If X is a discrete random variable, then its probability mass function is f_X:

$$f_X : \Omega' \to [0, 1] \quad \text{with} \quad f_X(x) = P(X = x).$$

The notation $P(X = x)$ reads: "The probability that the variable X takes the value x".

An important feature of probability mass functions is that all individual probabilities sum up to 1. For example, in the card-drawing example we get:

$$\frac{12}{32} + \frac{4}{32} + \frac{4}{32} + \frac{4}{32} + \frac{4}{32} + \frac{4}{32} = 1.$$

The concept of a probability mass function and its relation to a (discrete) random variable is also illustrated in Fig. 2.1 using the Skat example: The random experiment consists of randomly drawing a card from the deck, and the set Ω includes all of its 32 possible outcomes. The set Ω' comprises the property of interest (the card values), that is, the numbers 0, 2, 3, 4, 10, and 11. The mapping from Ω to Ω' is the discrete random variable and it assigns one of the possible card values to each element of Ω. Moreover, each of these card values occurs with a certain probability. These probabilities are summarized in another set P, and the mapping from Ω' to P is the probability mass function: It assigns to each element of Ω' its probability of occurrence. In other words: If we know the probability mass function for a (discrete) random variable and then perform the random experiment once (i.e., draw one card), we know the probability of obtaining a certain value of the set Ω'. For example, a card value of 0 occurs with a probability of $p_0 = \frac{12}{32}$.

An important question to resolve at this point is: How do we actually obtain a probability mass function? Possible strategies include:

- Deriving the probability mass function from properties of the random experiment. This is the case in our card-drawing example when there is no reason to believe that certain cards will be drawn preferentially.
- "Estimating" the probability mass function by assessing the relative frequency of multiple empirical realizations.
- Deriving the probability mass function mathematically. This is the most common approach in inferential statistics.

2.1.3   Expected Value of Discrete Random Variables

An important concept concerning random variables is the expected value, which is somewhat similar to the mean of actual data (see Sect. 1.3.1). Put simply, the **expected value** of a random variable is something like the "mean value that the random experiment will yield in the long run, that is, across many trials." For this purpose, imagine that we were to repeat the random experiment of drawing a single card from a full deck infinitely many times—or at least very, very often. The mean of the card values drawn in this process of repetitions would then be the expected value of the corresponding random variable. More generally, we often do not know the expected value—it is therefore a theoretical construct based on the probability mass function of the random variable. If X is a discrete random variable, then its expected value $E(X)$ is:

$$E(X) = \sum_{x \in \Omega'} x \cdot P(X = x). \tag{2.1}$$

Occasionally, the expected value $E(X)$ of a random variable X is also denoted as μ_X (read: "mu X"). Formula 2.1 means: We multiply all elements from Ω' with their probability of occurrence and sum up these products. In the card drawing example, the elements of Ω' are the card values 0, 2, 3, 4, 10, and 11, and their respective probabilities of occurrence are $p = \frac{12}{32}$ and $p = \frac{4}{32}$. The expected value of the discrete random variable X that assigns a particular card value to each draw is thus:

$$E(X) = 0 \cdot \frac{12}{32} + 2 \cdot \frac{4}{32} + 3 \cdot \frac{4}{32} + 4 \cdot \frac{4}{32} + 10 \cdot \frac{4}{32} + 11 \cdot \frac{4}{32} = \frac{120}{32} = 3.75.$$

In other words, if we repeat the process of randomly drawing a card for an infinite number of times and then compute the mean of all obtained card values, it would be 3.75. Two *important properties of the expected value* are:

- The expected value of a discrete random variable needs not be an element of Ω'.
- If we do not go all the way up to infinity, but consider a finite number of repetitions of the random experiment instead (e.g., ten trials of drawing a single card from a full deck), then calculating the mean based on this sample will usually not correspond exactly to the expected value. However, it tends to approach the expected value, the more often we repeat the random experiment (see also Sect. 3.3).

2.1.4   Variance of Discrete Random Variables

We had mentioned above that the expected value of a random variable is approximately equal to the mean if we were to repeat the random experiment many times. Similarly, there is also a variance for random variables. This variance corresponds to the expected mean squared deviation from the expected value. If X is a discrete random variable, then its variance σ_X^2 is:

$$\sigma_X^2 = E[(X - E(X))^2]. \tag{2.2}$$

Sometimes, the variance of a random variable σ_X^2 is also denoted as $V(X)$. The square root of the variance is called standard deviation σ_X ("sigma"; see Formula 1.4 in the case of descriptive statistics).

2.2   Continuous Random Variables

In psychology (and other empirical sciences), we often measure variables such as height, reaction time, etc. In principle, these variables can take an infinite number of values, and Ω' therefore contains an infinite number of elements. In such a case, we speak of a **continuous random variable**. Although the concept is similar to that of discrete random variables, there are some important differences regarding the probability of individual values and the probability for ranges of values.

2.2.1 Probability Density Functions

In case of discrete random variables, the probability mass function is used to specify the probability of occurrence for each element of Ω'. In case of continuous random variables, however, Ω' has infinitely many elements, and thus—paradoxically—the probability of observing any individual value becomes zero. However, we can specify the probability of observing a value within a certain range. We thus do not speak about probability mass functions in this case but of a **probability density function** for continuous random variables. Before taking a look at actual probability density functions, we first consider an important property: probability density functions are *normalized*, that is, their total area under the curve is exactly 1.[2] Mathematically speaking, this property means that the integral of a probability density function $f(x)$ calculated from $-\infty$ to $+\infty$ equals 1:

$$\int_{-\infty}^{+\infty} f(x)dx = 1.$$

Because of this property, we can interpret areas under the probability density function as probabilities. If we know the probability density function for a given continuous random variable, and if we draw a single element $\omega \in \Omega$ then a first obvious conclusion is: The value of Ω' assigned to this element ω falls into the range from $-\infty$ to $+\infty$ with probability 1.

More interesting are more narrowly defined ranges of values. Figure 2.3 shows an example of a probability density function of a continuous random variable X. We now draw a single $\omega \in \Omega$. What is the probability of observing an element, for which the random variable X assigns a value between -1 and 0? Since, as we said, we can interpret areas as probabilities, the probability we are looking for corresponds to the gray area in Fig. 2.3, and its value is the integral of the probability density function from -1 to 0:

$$p(-1 \leq x \leq 0) = \int_{-1}^{0} f(x)dx.$$

In Depth 2.3: Alternate Uses
Of course, we can use probability density functions the other way around: If we know the probability density function of a continuous random variable, we can determine a point k that cuts off a certain proportion, say 5%, of the total area under the probability density function (e.g., on the right tail). This can be done by means

(continued)

---

[2] This is similar to the probability mass function for discrete random variables, where the individual probabilities always sum up to 1 as discussed in Sect. 2.1.2.

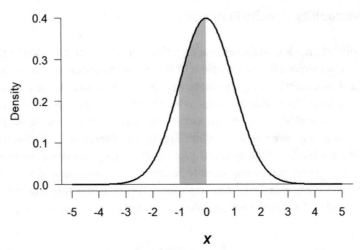

Fig. 2.3 Example of a probability density function of a continuous random variable X. The gray area corresponds to the probability that the random variable takes a value between -1 and 0

of integral calculus, and the solution for k can be calculated using the following integral:

$$\int_k^\infty f(x)dx = 0.05.$$

2.2.2 Expected Value and Variance of Continuous Random Variables

To calculate the expected value of discrete random variables (Formula 2.1), we made use of the probability of observing individual values. Unfortunately, calculating the expected value of continuous random variables this way is not possible, because individual values have a probability of 0 in the continuous case. The expected value of a continuous random variable X is thus defined as:

$$E(X) = \int_{-\infty}^{+\infty} x \cdot f(x)dx.$$

The variance σ_X^2 or $V(X)$ corresponds to that of discrete random variables (Formula 2.2).

2.3   The Normal Distribution

Several specific probability density functions are commonplace in many applications of inferential statistics. In this book, we will use various probability density functions based on the so-called t-distribution (Chap. 5) or the F-distribution (Chap. 8).

First, however, we will discuss the most widespread and important probability density function: the normal distribution. Strictly speaking, the **normal distribution** (also called the Gaussian distribution) is a whole family of distributions with the characteristic shape of a bell curve. The exact shape of a normal distribution depends on two parameters: its expected value μ and its variance σ^2. If a random variable X is normally distributed, this is written as:

$$X \sim N(\mu, \sigma^2).$$

In such abbreviated notations for the distribution of a random variable, the name of that random variable is always given first. The tilde ($\sim$) means "is distributed" and is followed by the type of distribution (and its parameters). Here, N is the usual abbreviation for a normal distribution, and its probability density function is given by:

$$f(x) = \frac{1}{\sqrt{2\pi\sigma^2}} \cdot e^{-\frac{(x-\mu)^2}{2\sigma^2}}.$$

Figure 2.4 shows four examples of normal distributions with different parameters. It also showcases the relationship between parameter values and the resulting form of the normal distribution: The expected value μ corresponds to the x-coordinate of the "highest point" (peak; compare the solid curve with the dotted curve), whereas the variance determines

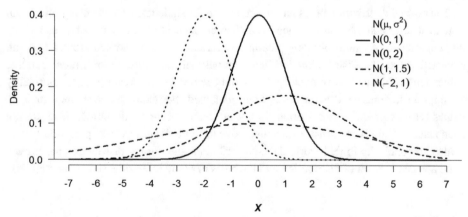

Fig. 2.4 Examples of normal distributions with different parameters. $N(0, 1)$ is also called the standard normal distribution

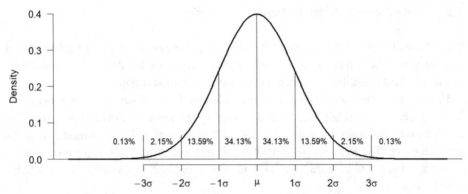

Fig. 2.5 Probability density function of a normal distribution with area proportions highlighted. The points -1σ and 1σ represent the inflection points of the (standard) normal distribution

how "wide" the curve is (compare the solid curve with the dashed and the dotted-dashed curve). A special case is the distribution $N(0, 1)$, which is also called **standard normal distribution**. Any normal distribution can be transformed into a standard normal distribution by the z-transformation, and the standard normal distribution is available in many statistics books and computer programs.

Figure 2.4 also shows one of the most important properties of normal distributions: They are symmetric in that they look like mirror images on either side of the expected value. At the same time, the largest proportion of their area lies near the expected value, and this proportion becomes smaller the further we move away from the expected value. Furthermore, an interesting aspect of all normal distributions is that their standard deviation can be interpreted descriptively: The range ± 1 standard deviation around the expected value houses 68% of the area, that is, $P(\mu - \sigma \leq x \leq \mu + \sigma) \approx 0.68$ (see Fig. 2.5).

The normal distribution plays an important role for statistics, because many inferential statistical tests assume that the measured characteristic is normally distributed. Indeed, the major share of values of many measurable variables is concentrated around a certain expected value, the distribution is often symmetrical, and furthermore, more extreme values tend to occur less frequently. We should remember, however, that the normality assumption for measured variables is often idealized. For example, very small or large values (close to $-\infty$ or $+\infty$) often do not or cannot occur at all. Often, there are not even negative values and strictly speaking—due to limited measurement precision—there is also no continuity in real-world data. Nevertheless, the normal distribution has proven to be a versatile form of distribution and the basis of many inferential statistical methods.

Introduction to Inferential Statistics 2: Population and Parameter Estimation

3

This chapter aims to provide an understanding of why we need inferential statistics. To this end, we will first turn to the important distinction between population and sample before moving on to the topic of parameter estimation. The following chapters will build on this reasoning by applying this logic to the most common procedures in statistical inference.

3.1 Sample vs. Population

3.1.1 The Problem

The distinction of population and sample is at the core of inferential statistics. Usually, we are interested in inferring general conclusions about a population, but we only have a sample from that population.

We will approach this distinction with an exemplary research question that we will revisit also in later chapters: Are certain motor activities, such as rolling cigars, performed more easily in daylight or with artificial lighting? To answer this question, we conduct a fictitious study and have one group of participants roll cigars for an hour in daylight, and a second group of participants roll cigars in artificial light. The dependent variable is the amount of cigars rolled during this time.[1] Table 3.1 shows the fictitious results of the participants in this experiment.

---

[1] Indeed, several psychological theories such as the power law of motor learning have been demonstrated using cigar rolling as an example (Crossman 1959; Fitts and Posner 1967; see Rosenbaum and Janczyk 2019, for more information on Crossman).

© Springer-Verlag GmbH Germany, part of Springer Nature 2023
M. Janczyk, R. Pfister, *Understanding Inferential Statistics*,
https://doi.org/10.1007/978-3-662-66786-6_3

Table 3.1 Results of the exemplary experiment. Data represent the number of cigars rolled in one hour by each of ten participants working either under daylight or with artificial lighting

	1	2	3	4	5	6	7	8	9	10
Daylight	21	20	19	26	18	21	22	23	23	24
Artificial light	18	16	18	19	22	16	17	18	19	24

We can now compute means and variances for both samples as sample statistics (see Formulas 1.2 and 1.3):

$$M_{\text{daylight}} = 21.7 \quad \text{and} \quad S^2_{\text{daylight}} = 5.21,$$

$$M_{\text{artificial light}} = 18.7 \quad \text{and} \quad S^2_{\text{artificial light}} = 5.81.$$

At first glance, we see that the mean value when working under daylight is higher than when working under artificial light. We might thus be inclined to conclude that performance under daylight seems to be generally higher.

On closer inspection, however, we might hesitate to draw strong conclusions. After all, there are many more than ten people in this world and we could have examined each of these persons under daylight or artificial light. The set of all these persons that we could have investigated in theory is usually called the population. We cannot rule out that we happened to have several people in the daylight sample who are particularly good at rolling cigars anyway. In any case, it is theoretically possible that we could have obtained a completely opposite result with two other (random) samples.

A conclusion that is "absolutely correct" logically requires knowing the population means—in most cases, this alternative will be impossible to achieve in its strict sense. In the example, we would have to test all persons in the world, including all those who have ever existed or will exist in the future.

Whenever we want to draw general conclusions, we are therefore in the situation that we cannot know the values that we are actually interested in, that is, the mean values of the populations. All we can know is based on the samples at hand. The basic question of inferential statistics therefore is: How can we infer statements about the population on the basis of a sample? In a first step, we will try to estimate the "population mean" as precisely as possible based on the available sample (Sect. 3.2). In Sect. 3.3 we will then address the question of what a "good" estimate is in a statistical sense. Finally, in Sect. 3.4 we turn to the estimation of the population variance. The procedure discussed in this chapter is one of the foundations of inferential statistics and is known as parameter estimation.

3.1.2 Sample Statistics and Population Parameters

The following steps build on the critical distinction between sample and population. To stress this difference, statisticians use a distinct notation to refer to concepts on these two levels: The unknown values on the population level are usually called **population parameters** and are denoted by Greek letters. In contrast, values that we can calculate from a sample—the **sample statistics**—are denoted by Latin letters (see also Table 3.2).

Figure 3.1 illustrates the interplay of sample and population: For a normally distributed variable (in this case: IQ), there is a mean μ in the population and a corresponding variance σ^2 (or standard deviation σ). During sampling, individual elements (usually people) are randomly drawn from the population and we can calculate sample statistics from the resulting sample. **Parameter estimation** uses these statistics to make inferences about the unknown population parameters. We therefore turn to the question of how the population parameter μ can be optimally estimated from a sample and then continue by discussing general rules of what makes a good estimator.

Table 3.2 Mean and variance as sample statistics and population parameters

Sample statistic	Population parameter
$M_X,\ \bar{X}$	$\mu,\ E(X)$
S_X^2	σ_X^2

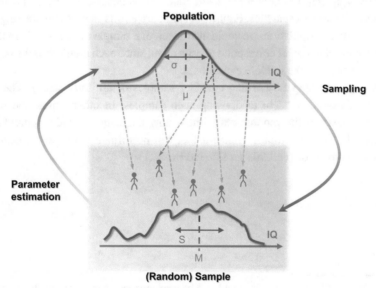

Fig. 3.1 The distinction of population and sample, and the interplay of sampling and parameter estimation

3.2   The Population Parameter μ

Intuitively, it seems reasonable to assume that the mean of a sample is well suited for estimating the population mean μ.[2] For now let us simply assume that an estimator for μ is "good" if its value is likely to be close to the population mean μ.

In order to approach the best possible estimate of μ, let us consider an example population. This population consists of only five persons for each of whom we know the value on a variable X:

$$x_1 = 2, \quad x_2 = 4, \quad x_3 = 6, \quad x_4 = 6, \quad x_5 = 7.$$

Because we know the entire population, we can easily use the formulas for the mean and variance (Formulas 1.2 and 1.3) to calculate the two population parameters μ and σ^2 in this case as:[3]

$$\mu = 5 \quad \text{and} \quad \sigma_X^2 = 3.2. \tag{3.1}$$

In Chap. 2 we stated that randomly drawing a person (from a population) can be regarded as a random experiment. This chapter also introduced the concept of random variables, that is, mappings that assign to each element of a set Ω an element of a second set Ω'.

The following step requires some abstraction, but is necessary for understanding the mechanics of inferential statistics. Figure 3.2 summarizes this step. When drawing a single individual from the population, we could also speak of a sample of size $n = 1$. In this case, the population and the set Ω correspond to each other, since each member of the population can be the outcome of the random experiment.

We now go one step further and consider samples of arbitrary size n. The random experiment is now equivalent to drawing such samples. In other words, the set of all possible outcomes of the random experiment now no longer includes individuals, but it includes all possible samples of size n that can be formed from the elements of the population. We therefore call this set Ω^n (see Box 3.1).

---

[2] Other measures of central tendency could also be used in theory, such as the mode or the median. However, as we will see later, it is mainly the arithmetic mean that meets common quality criteria (see Sect. 3.3).

[3] Remember that this is an unrealistic situation in most cases: If we actually knew the population parameters, we would no longer need parameter estimation or inferential statistics. We could then rely on descriptive statistics alone to arrive at perfectly correct statements about the population.

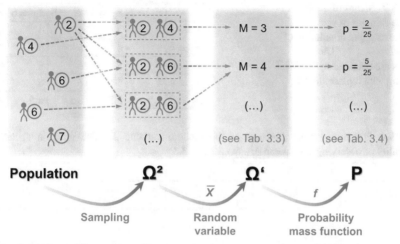

Fig. 3.2 Illustration of the steps involved in estimating the parameter μ. Starting from a set of five individuals, we draw (with replacement) all possible samples of size $n = 2$, which in turn form the set Ω^2. A random variable assigns to these samples their means; the possible means are therefore elements of the set Ω'. Finally, the probability mass function defines the probability of observing each possible mean value

---

In Depth 3.1: The Random Variable $\bar{X}$

In formal terms, the random variable $\bar{X}$ can be described as follows:

$$\bar{X} : \Omega^n \to \mathbb{R} \quad \text{with} \quad \underbrace{(\omega_1, \dots, \omega_n)}_{n\text{-tuple}} \to \underbrace{\frac{1}{n} \sum_{i=1}^{n} X_{\omega_i}}_{M}.$$

We thus define a mapping $\bar{X}$ from a set Ω^n (where n indicates the sample size) to the set of real numbers. The set Ω is the population, and the elements of the set Ω^n are so-called n-tuples, which in turn consist of elements ω_i from Ω—a sample of elements from the population. The assignment rule holds that the mapping assigns to each of these n-tuples the mean M of its components ω_i.

We first consider the simple case of sample size $n = 2$, that is, the set Ω^2 contains all possible samples of size $n = 2$ that can be drawn from the example population described above. A random variable now assigns to each of these samples the mean of its two elements, and we therefore call the random variable $\bar{X}$. The mean is a real number, so the second set Ω' (the set of possible means of the samples) is a subset of $\mathbb{R}$.

Table 3.3 Means of all 25 possible samples of size $n = 2$ from the example population of persons $x_1, \ldots, x_5$. The samples are obtained by sampling with replacement

	$x_1 = 2$	$x_2 = 4$	$x_3 = 6$	$x_4 = 6$	$x_5 = 7$
$x_1 = 2$	2	3	4	4	4.5
$x_2 = 4$	3	4	5	5	5.5
$x_3 = 6$	4	5	6	6	6.5
$x_4 = 6$	4	5	6	6	6.5
$x_5 = 7$	4.5	5.5	6.5	6.5	7

Table 3.4 Probability mass function of the random variable $\bar{X}$. The function specifies the probability of observing each mean M_x from Table 3.3

M_x	2	3	4	4.5	5	5.5	6	6.5	7
$P(\bar{X} = M_x)$	$\frac{1}{25}$	$\frac{2}{25}$	$\frac{5}{25}$	$\frac{2}{25}$	$\frac{4}{25}$	$\frac{2}{25}$	$\frac{4}{25}$	$\frac{4}{25}$	$\frac{1}{25}$

The means of all 25 possible samples of size $n = 2$ from the population are given in Table 3.3. It is important to note that we have sampled *with replacement*, that is, one and the same person may be drawn repeatedly and may therefore appear twice in a sample; we will come back to the implications of this later on.

If we further assume that all possible samples are equally probable (i.e., $p = \frac{1}{25}$), we can easily determine the corresponding probability mass function, which gives the probability that the random variable $\bar{X}$ takes a certain mean value M_X (see Table 3.4).[4]

Thus, we now have all we need to determine the parameters of the random variable $\bar{X}$ (see Formulas 2.1 and 2.2):

$$E(\bar{X}) = 5 \quad \text{and} \quad \sigma^2_{\bar{X}} = 1.6.$$

Comparing these values with the parameters of the population (Formula 3.1), one might assume:

$$E(\bar{X}) = \mu \quad \text{and} \quad \sigma^2_{\bar{X}} = \frac{\sigma^2_X}{n}, \tag{3.2}$$

where n denotes the size of the samples used, that is, $n = 2$ in the example. In fact, this conjecture is also true in the general case when the original variable under consideration, X, is normally distributed in the population with some expected value μ and a variance σ^2_X, that is, if $X \sim N(\mu, \sigma^2_X)$. The formal proof of this fact can be found in the online

---

[4] Because there is only a finite number of possible means in this example (i.e., the set Ω' is finitely large), $\bar{X}$ is a discrete random variable.

material. Before we proceed with deriving general concepts for parameter estimation, we would like to revisit two aspects of the preceding argument:

- First, we assumed that each sample is drawn with the same probability. This assumption is necessary to determine the probability mass function of the random variable $\bar{X}$, which, in turn, is necessary to calculate the expected value and variance of the random variable. Note, however, that this is an assumption. Whether this assumption is true for a given empirical study is a different question altogether. To meet this assumption as closely as possible, it is therefore important that the samples are *drawn randomly* (at least as randomly as possible) and that certain samples are not favored.
- Second, in our example, we have drawn 25 possible samples of size $n = 2$. Strictly speaking, however, the sample (2, 2), for example, should not exist at all, because there is only one person with the value 2 and one and the same person should not be in a sample twice in reality. In the example in Table 3.3 sampling was thus *with replacement*. There are two main reasons for this procedural choice: (1) All computations would become much more complicated if sampling without replacement, and (2) the deviation compared to sampling without replacement is negligible for large populations and usual sample sizes.

If we now were to draw all samples of the sizes n with $n \in \{3, 4, 5\}$ from the example population, and if we defined analogous random variables as for the case $n = 2$, then these random variables would also have the expected value of 5 (according to Formula 3.2), and their variance would become successively smaller with larger n. Finally, we could observe that the means of the samples are distributed in a particular way. This observation is important and deserves closer inspection.

Figure 3.3 shows the relative frequencies of the means of 3000 samples of size $n = 5$ drawn from the example population (again sampling with replacement). The visual impression suggests that these means follow a normal distribution, and means around the value 5 seem to be particularly common. Remember, this value corresponds to the population mean and thus to the expected value of the random variable $\bar{X}$. Means that are far from 5 occur less frequently. In fact, the conjecture of normal distribution is true if we again assume that the original variable X is normally distributed in the population and the individual samples of size n are drawn independently from each other. Under these conditions, a random variable $\bar{X}$, assigning the sample mean to samples of size n, is normally distributed with an expected value $E(\bar{X}) = \mu$ and a variance $\sigma_{\bar{X}}^2 = \frac{\sigma_X^2}{n}$.

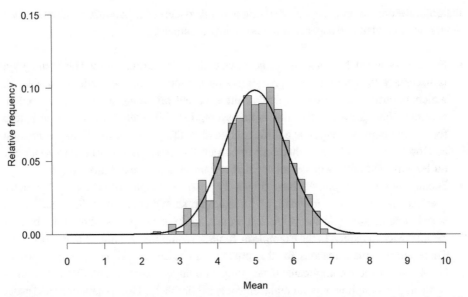

Fig. 3.3 Relative frequencies of the sample means from 3000 samples of size $n = 5$ (sampled with replacement), which were drawn from the example population

In Depth 3.2: The Random Variable $\bar{X}$

In formal terms, we would express this fact as follows: Let $X \sim N(\mu, \sigma^2)$ and be $X_1, \ldots, X_n$ n independent realizations of X. Then, for the random variable $\bar{X}$ holds:

$$\bar{X} \sim N\left(\mu, \frac{\sigma^2}{n}\right). \tag{3.3}$$

One aspect of these derivations might feel familiar, as it already appeared in the previous chapters. The square root of the variance of the random variable $\bar{X}$,

$$\sqrt{\frac{\sigma_{\bar{X}}^2}{n}} = \frac{\sigma_X}{\sqrt{n}},$$

is what we have introduced in Chap. 1 as the **standard error of the mean** (see Formula 1.5).

In summary, the expected value of the distribution of means, that is, of the random variable $\bar{X}$, is equal to the population parameter μ. These mean values are also normally distributed, so that the majority of the values of $\bar{X}$ is concentrated around μ. The mean thus seems to be a good estimator for the population parameter μ. Even though the two will not be identical in most practical scenarios, using the mean as an estimator is actually the best we can do.

3.3   Desired Properties of Parameter Estimators

In addition to the mean, we could use any sample statistic as an estimator for a population parameter of interest. However, each statistic should meet certain requirements to be considered a good estimator. To operationalize what we have considered "good" in case of the mean, we now introduce two (most important) **desired properties of parameter estimators**.

- **Unbiasedness:** Estimators are considered unbiased if the expected value of a random variable assigning this estimator to the elements of Ω^n (e.g., samples) is equal to the to-be-estimated population parameter. Thus, unbiasedness means that the estimator does not under- or overestimate the parameter systematically.
  We have already encountered one example of an unbiased estimator: the (arithmetic) mean. The expected value of a random variable $\bar{X}$, which assigns samples their means, corresponds exactly to the population parameter μ. Hence, M is an unbiased estimator of μ (the formal proof of this property can be found in the online material).
- **Consistency:** Estimators are considered consistent if increasing the sample size increases the probability that the estimator is close to the population parameter.
  We have already seen that the variance of the distribution of the means becomes smaller with increasing sample size n, that is, the (normal) distribution becomes narrower. Intuitively, this suggests that, as the sample size increases, the estimation of μ with M becomes more accurate. Thus, the probability of obtaining a mean close to the population parameter increases with sample size n. In other words: We can assume that M is a consistent estimator for μ—and this is indeed the case.

In Depth 3.3: Formal Definition of Unbiasedness and Consistency
The concepts of unbiasedness and consistency can of course be expressed formally:

- **Unbiasedness:** Let T be an estimator for the population parameter τ (a lowercase tau). Then T is an unbiased estimator for τ if

$$E(T) = \tau.$$

(continued)

- **Consistency:** Let τ be a population parameter and T_n a sequence of estimators, where n is the sample size. T_n is a consistent estimator for τ if the following relation is true for any $\epsilon > 0$ ($\epsilon \in \mathbb{R}$):

$$P(|T_n - \tau| \geq \epsilon) \to 0 \qquad \text{for } n \to \infty.$$

3.4   The Population Parameter σ^2

So far, we have considered the population parameter μ and we know that M is an unbiased and consistent estimator for it. We now consider the population variance σ_X^2. Intuitively, the sample variance S_X^2 might be the appropriate estimator in this case.

Just as in the case of μ, we now consider a random variable S_X^2 that assigns to each sample of size n its sample variance.

In Depth 3.4: The Random Variable S_X^2

We can also describe this random variable formally:

$$S_X^2 : \Omega^n \to \mathbb{R} \qquad \text{with} \qquad (\omega_1, \ldots, \omega_n) \to \underbrace{\frac{\sum_{i=1}^n (X_{\omega_i} - M_\omega)^2}{n}}_{S_X^2}.$$

Similar to what we did for the mean with the random variable $\bar{X}$, each n-tuple (i.e., each sample of the elements ω_i from Ω) is assigned the variance of its elements.

Now the question is: Is S_X^2 an unbiased estimator for σ_X^2? If this was the case, then $E(S_X^2) = \sigma_X^2$ should be true. Calculating the expected value of S_X^2 (see the online material), yields a different result, however:

$$E(S_X^2) = \frac{n-1}{n} \sigma_X^2.$$

Apparently, this result does not meet the definition of unbiasedness: S_X^2 is therefore *not* an unbiased estimator for σ_X^2. Unbiasedness would only be realized if the factor $\frac{n-1}{n}$ disappears. This can be achieved by multiplying with $\frac{n}{n-1}$ and we now consider, as a second try, a different random variable $\hat{S}_X^2$, which no longer assigns each sample its sample variance S_X^2, but a **corrected sample variance** $\hat{S}_X^2 = \frac{n}{n-1} S_X^2$. The expected value of this random variable is in fact σ_X^2—it is therefore the unbiased estimator we are looking for (see also the online material). Moreover, this corrected sample variance is also a consistent estimator.

When defining the sample variance in Sect. 1.3, we pointed out that, instead of dividing by n, some books introduce the variance by dividing by $n - 1$. We can now see why this is sometimes done, as slightly restructuring the corrected sample variance yields:

$$\hat{S}_X^2 = \frac{n}{n-1} S_X^2 = \frac{n}{n-1} \cdot \frac{1}{n} \sum_{i=1}^{n} (x_i - M_X)^2 = \frac{1}{n-1} \sum_{i=1}^{n} (x_i - M_X)^2.$$

Thus, if we divide by $n - 1$, we instantly get the corrected sample variance, and thus an unbiased estimator of the population variance. Three concluding remarks on this distinction:

- In this book, we consistently distinguish between the (descriptive) sample variance S_X^2 and the corrected sample variance $\hat{S}_X^2 = \frac{n}{n-1} S_X^2$ (as an unbiased estimator of the population variance σ_X^2). Thus, it is always important to pay attention to which variance is used in the formulas.

  In many statistical programs, this is not done (see Sect. 1.3). The descriptive statistics functions in SPSS for instance return the corrected sample variance as output and the same applies to the corresponding functions var() and sd() in R.
- We have referred to the appropriate estimator for the population variance as $\hat{S}_X^2$. Sometimes we will use the notation $\hat{\sigma}_X^2$ instead, because in statistics the "hat" above a symbol denotes an estimator for the corresponding parameter.
- In later chapters, we will use $\hat{S}_X$ as an estimator for the population standard deviation σ_X. This is not a new quantity, but $\hat{S}_X = \sqrt{\hat{S}_X^2}$.

Hypothesis Testing and Significance

4

In Chap. 3 we have introduced the concept of parameter estimation and we have discovered suitable estimators for the population mean μ and the population variance σ^2. Now we have all we need to actually test hypotheses about such parameters. We will do so by using the logic of so-called null hypothesis significance testing. When conducting such hypothesis tests, we first transform substantive hypotheses into a statistical formulation relating to population parameters. We then decide between two mutually exclusive hypotheses based on the result of a significance test.

We will begin with a brief overview of different ways to classify statistical hypotheses, and then introduce the logic of significance testing based on a hands-on example. This logic is also the basis for all the test procedures discussed in the further chapters (t-tests, analyses of variance, . . .).

4.1 Substantive and Statistical Hypotheses

The expected outcome of a study will typically speak towards a **substantive hypothesis**. We have already seen an example of this in Sect. 3.1.1. There we had asked whether more cigars can be rolled in daylight or artificial light.

In statistical hypothesis testing, substantive hypotheses must be converted into statistical formulations that make statements about population parameters. **Statistical hypotheses** can be formulated about differences or about correlations, and both can be directional or non-directional. Last, but certainly not least, there is the crucial distinction between null and alternative hypotheses.

© Springer-Verlag GmbH Germany, part of Springer Nature 2023
M. Janczyk, R. Pfister, *Understanding Inferential Statistics*,
https://doi.org/10.1007/978-3-662-66786-6_4

4.1.1 Classification of Statistical Hypotheses

Difference hypotheses predict a difference between two (or more) conditions or of one condition and a fixed value. Referring to the example from Sect. 3.1.1, a difference hypothesis would be: *"The numbers of cigars rolled per hour differ between daylight and artificial lighting conditions."* In contrast, **correlation hypotheses** postulate relationships or associations between variables. An example would be: *"The more experience a person has with rolling cigars, the more cigars they can roll per hour."*

Because statistical hypotheses relate to population parameters, we try to answer questions such as: Do the corresponding parameters of the populations differ, that is, $\mu_{\text{daylight}} \neq \mu_{\text{artificial light}}$? Although we will again rely on samples to answer this question, of course, we are actually less interested in the question of whether $M_{\text{daylight}} \neq M_{\text{artificial light}}$. Even if two population means are the same, two sample means will usually differ (we will illustrate this in Sect. 4.2.1).

Both difference and correlation hypotheses can be non-directional or directional. **Non-directional hypotheses** are formulated, when there is no reasonable assumption about the direction of the difference or the relationship. The formulation above was already an example of this: *"The numbers of cigars rolled per hour differ between daylight and artificial lighting conditions."*—without predicting which condition comes with better performance. If there were theoretical reasons to assume a direction, we could also formulate a **directed hypothesis**: *"More cigars are rolled per hour in daylight than with artificial light."* Both exemplary hypotheses are called **non-specific** or **inexact hypotheses**. A **specific** or **exact hypothesis**, on the other hand, states an exact difference between two populations. This can again either involve a non-directional or a directional statement. For example, *"The number of cigars rolled in daylight and in artificial light differ by exactly three cigars per hour"* (non-directional) or *"Three cigars more can be rolled per hour in daylight than in artificial light"* (directional).

4.1.2 Alternative and Null Hypothesis

As just mentioned, we are usually not interested in the samples as such, but in the populations behind them—and the hypotheses therefore make statements about population parameters. As an example, let us consider the *non-directional* substantive hypothesis *"The numbers of cigars rolled per hour differ between daylight and artificial lighting conditions"*. Its statistical formulation—that is, a formulation targeting the corresponding population means—then is:

$$H_1 : \mu_{\text{daylight}} \neq \mu_{\text{artificial light}}.$$

This so-called **alternative hypothesis H_1** is contrasted with the **null hypothesis H_0** that asserts the logical opposite:

$$H_0 : \mu_{\text{daylight}} = \mu_{\text{artificial light}}.$$

Formulating such a pair of hypotheses is the starting point of any hypothesis test. In case of a *directional* hypothesis about differences, such a pair would be:

$$H_0 : \mu_{\text{daylight}} \leq \mu_{\text{artificial light}} \quad \text{and} \quad H_1 : \mu_{\text{daylight}} > \mu_{\text{artificial light}}.$$

The null hypothesis $\mu_A = \mu_B$ is also **specific**: It is satisfied if and only if the two μs are identical. The alternative hypothesis is usually **non-specific**: There is an infinite number of possible values of the two μs for which it would be true. We will come back to this issue in Chap. 7 when discussing the concept of *statistical power*. In what follows, we will focus on the case of a specific null hypothesis, since this type of hypothesis is the central starting point in null hypothesis testing. The fact that the null hypothesis for a directional alternative hypothesis does not state equality, but "less than or equal to", as above, is necessary because the two hypotheses must cover all theoretically possible patterns that might exist in the population.

4.2 The Idea of the Significance Test

A common significance test probes for differences between two so-called independent samples.[1] In the following section, we cover the general procedure for this case. In the next chapter, we will then transfer and apply this logic to the corresponding "real" significance test, the *t*-test for two independent samples.

4.2.1 A Fictitious Situation. . .

Let us assume the following situation: We have formulated a directional alternative hypothesis stating that the mean of a given variable in one population A is larger than in a second population B:

$$H_0 : \mu_A \leq \mu_B \quad \text{and} \quad H_1 : \mu_A > \mu_B.$$

These hypotheses cover all possible constellations of μ_A and μ_B in line with the requirements for statistical hypotheses introduced above. Now, the following considerations are

---

[1] We will return to the distinction between dependent and independent samples in Sect. 5.3.

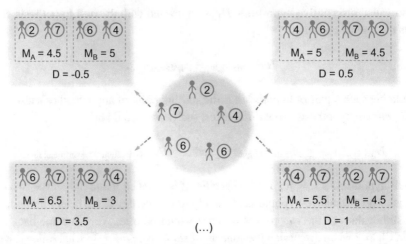

Fig. 4.1 Two samples of size $n = 2$ are drawn from a population of (five) people with a certain measurable characteristic. We can now calculate the mean value for both samples, and $D = M_A - M_B$ indicates the difference in means. Although both samples come from the same population, the mean values usually differ, that is, $D \neq 0$

based on the exact formulation of the null hypothesis, that is, on $H_0 : \mu_A = \mu_B$. In this case, the populations are identical with respect to their population mean, so that we can simply speak of the same population in this regard.

For the sake of simplicity, let us imagine that we know the population(s) and we again use the example from Sect. 3.2. In a fictitious study, two samples are drawn from populations A and B, and the sample sizes are identical, that is, $n_A = n_B$. Because we assume H_0 to be true in the population, both samples are effectively drawn from a single population. If we then calculate the sample means M_A and M_B, it is still highly unlikely that $M_A = M_B$, because both means are generated by random sampling. Thus, in general $M_A \neq M_B$; in other words, almost always will we observe a non-zero difference $D = M_A - M_B \neq 0$. Figure 4.1 illustrates this point with four exemplary draws of two samples of size $n = 2$.

4.2.2   . . . and the Logic of the Significance Test

In the following, we will use the described situation to develop the idea of **significance testing**. First, suppose we knew the probability of observing each possible value of D if H_0 were true, that is, when both samples are drawn from the same population. If we now observe a single, empirical D-value from a single study and see that the probability of observing this value (or even more extreme values) is "very low", then we doubt our original assumption, that is, we question the validity of H_0. Instead, because there is only one other option, we assume that the H_1 is true.[2]

But what exactly do we mean with a "very low" probability? Let us agree that we consider a probability to be "very low" if it is smaller than 5%, and let us call this probability the **significance level** α (i.e., $\alpha = 0.05$). At first glance, this value seems rather arbitrary (and arbitrary it is), but scientists have become accustomed to the convention of using a value of 5% or 1%.

As a last hurdle, we now need to answer the following question: What values do occur for D if we assume the H_0 to be true? And further: Which values or value ranges occur rather frequently and which only rarely? This, of course, must be established so that we can estimate whether our single, empirical D or more extreme values are "very unlikely".

To approach the answer, we again consider a simulation: Let us imagine that we draw our two samples of size $n = 2$ not only four times (as in Fig. 4.1), but we instead draw samples of size $n = 5$ for 2000 times (with replacement). For each iteration, we then compute the two means of the samples and their difference D. The left panel of Fig. 4.2 shows the outcome of such a simulation. (We will discuss the right part of the figure later.)

Two features of the results catch the eye (Fig. 4.2, left panel): (1) Values around 0 seem to occur most frequently, and (2) the frequencies seem to be distributed symmetrically around this value. Overall, the distribution even looks approximately like a normal distribution. Before we continue with sketching the decision logic, we consider again the alternative hypothesis $H_1 : \mu_A > \mu_B$ formulated above. This means that an empirical result only speaks in favor of our hypothesis if $M_A > M_B$ or if $D = M_A - M_B > 0$. In the left panel of Fig. 4.2, some areas of the difference values D are colored red, others are colored green: Red are those values that together account for (about) 5% of all difference values at the right end of the whole distribution. In the example, this corresponds to the values $D \geq 2.25$. This value is what is also called a "critical value": Values that are larger than or equal to the critical value occur with a maximum probability of 0.05 when assuming the null hypothesis to be true. Conversely, the remaining values marked in green add up to 95%. With this knowledge at hand, we now consider two exemplary values for D:

- $D = 1$: In the left panel of Fig. 4.2, we can see that this value or larger values are rather frequent when the H_0 is true. Conversely, such a likely result provides little reason to doubt the initial assumption that the H_0 is true. We would therefore continue to assume that there is no difference between μ_A and μ_B.

---

[2] Considering the probability of observing either the measured value for D or more extreme values is useful and sometimes necessary for several reasons. For instance, if we had fine-grained measurements, the probability of a particular outcome is necessarily small (in case of continuous variables it is even 0), so that we cannot draw meaningful conclusions from the probability of a particular event. However, because more extreme—here: larger—values would also speak against the H_0, we assess the probability of the observed value or even more extreme data instead.

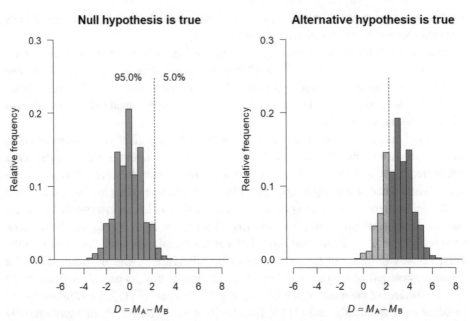

Fig. 4.2 Relative frequencies of differences in means when drawing two samples of size $n = 5$ from the population and repeating the process 2000 times. The left panel shows the results of a simulation that assumed the null hypothesis to be true (i.e., both samples were drawn from the example population), whereas the right panel shows a similar simulation when assuming the alternative hypothesis to be true (see text for more information)

- $D = 3$: In the left panel of Fig. 4.2, we see that this value or even larger values occur only rarely and are therefore very unlikely (their probability of occurring is less than 5%). In case of such an unlikely result, we have reasonable doubts about the assumption that the H_0 is true. We would then decide against assuming the H_0 and instead believe in the H_1—that is, assume that $\mu_A > \mu_B$. In such a case, we speak of a **significant result** of the test. Significant here means "clear" (Latin *significans:* clear, distinct).

4.2.3   Decisions and Decision Errors

Using the knowledge from the last section, we can now construct a fairly simple rule for deciding between the H_0 and the H_1:

If $D \geq$ "critical value", then we decide in favor of H_1 and reject H_0.

The critical value here depends solely on the value that we decide to use as α. For example, if we set $\alpha = 0.01$, we get a larger critical value than for $\alpha = 0.05$.

We can use another variant of a decision rule by calculating the probability p of observing a certain D-value or an even larger value. In the example, this probability can be determined as a relative frequency. An equivalent decision rule would therefore be:

> If $p \leq \alpha$, then we decide in favor of H_1 and reject H_0.

In the simulation underlying the left panel of Fig. 4.2, there were five instances with $D \geq 3$; this corresponds to a probability $p = P(D \geq 3) = \frac{5}{2000} = 0.0025$. The decision would therefore be identical for both rules (and in fact this is generally true).

We can already note a few additional points here, and we will get back to these points in the following chapters:

- For the simulation performed above (the one underlying the left panel of Fig. 4.2), we know that the H_0 was true, since we have drawn both samples from the same population. Improbable values—those in the red area—still occurred. They are very unlikely, but not impossible. In such a case, we would then decide for the H_1, and because we know that the H_0 was true, we would come to a wrong decision. That is: With the common criterion of $\alpha = 0.05$, in five out of 100 cases we would get a result that leads to a decision in favor of the H_1 if the H_0 is actually true in the population (see also the following Box 4.1). In this case, we speak of a Type I error (or α-error), and we will address the problem of such erroneous decisions in Chap. 7 in more detail.

In Depth 4.1: Interpreting Significance Levels
The interpretation "Five out of 100 results are significant, even if the H_0 is true." is intuitive, but it is actually somewhat simplified. A correct statement would read: Suppose the H_0 was true in the population and we applied the $\alpha = 0.05$ criterion. If we were then to conduct the same study an infinite number of times, we would get a significant result (i.e., a decision in favor of the H_1) in 5% of the repetitions.

- The value p from the above example gives the probability of the observed or even more extreme data (here: a larger D) when assuming that the H_0 is true. But what we actually want to know is something about the probability of one of the two hypotheses in light of the data. Statistical significance tests *cannot* provide this information, however.[3] The probability p (which is also the main output of many statistical programs) is formally a *conditional probability*:

---

[3] An approximation for this probability is provided by so-called Bayesian statistics. We will discuss the basics of these approaches in Chap. 12.

$$p = P(\text{data}|H_0).$$

This notation means "the probability of these (or more extreme) results given the H_0 is true". This probability should never be confused with the converse probability, that is, the "probability that the H_0 is true in light of the empirical data":

$$P(\text{data}|H_0) \neq P(H_0|\text{data}).$$

Thus, a significance test always provides only an indirect value on which to base the decision for one of the two statistical hypotheses. Never does a significance test allow us to make precise statements about the probability with which the two hypotheses are true.

So far, in the simulation and all following considerations, we had assumed that the H_0 is true and, accordingly, we have drawn both samples from the same population. We now consider the case when both samples come from different populations, that is, when the H_1 is true instead. The right panel of Fig. 4.2 visualizes this situation. For the underlying simulation, we again drew sample B from the population with the values 2, 4, 6, 6, and 7, but sample A now came from a population with the values 5, 7, 9, 9, and 10 (so we simply added 3 to each value). First, we can see that the resulting distribution has shifted to the right and frequent differences are now clustered around 3 (instead of 0). The dashed line again marks the value 2.25, which we determined to be the value "to the right of which" we would have 5% of the difference values if the H_0 is true (left panel of Fig. 4.2). It is clear from the right panel of Fig. 4.2 that if the H_1 is true, that is, if there is a difference in population means, a higher proportion of difference values is larger than or equal to 2.25. According to the decision rule that we introduced above, these are the difference values for which we decide in favor of the H_1. In other words: We determine a critical value under the assumption that the H_0 is true. However, the results of an empirical investigation are more likely to exceed this value if there is indeed a difference in population means (in the hypothesized direction). It is also clear, though, that we have also obtained difference values smaller than 2.25 in the simulation. In these cases, according to the decision rule, we would (continue to) assume that the H_0 is true. Hence, since we know in the simulation that the H_1 is true, we would again make a wrong decision. In such a case, we talk about a Type II error (or β-error). We will come back to the two possible decision errors in more detail in Chap. 7.

In summary, significance testing provides us with a simple and formalized rule to decide between the H_1 and the H_0. A key component of this decision rule is the so-called significance level, because it determines which observations we would like to treat as "very unlikely". This approach does not preclude wrong decisions, and decision errors

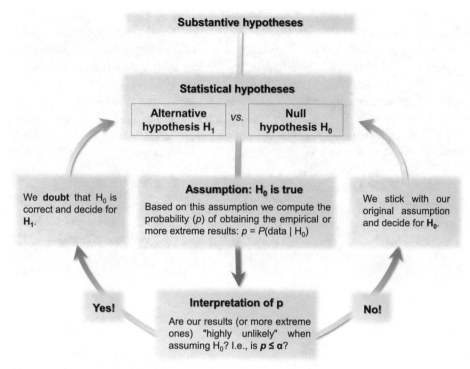

Fig. 4.3 Illustration of the decision procedure underlying null hypothesis significance testing

are explicitly included as a possible outcome. Across many studies, however, the logic of significance testing allows for controlling the likelihood of such erroneous decisions, and this stringent control over the average error rate is a decisive strength of these procedures. Moreover, the basic procedure of hypothesis testing is identical for all significance tests and we will encounter it again and again in the course of the next chapters. Fig. 4.3 summarizes the most important steps in this procedure.

In Depth 4.2: A Short History

Null hypothesis significance testing as it is commonly used today is actually a mixture of two concepts developed in the past century by Ronald A. Fisher on the one hand, as well as Jerzy Neyman and Egon S. Pearson on the other hand (see Gigerenzer and Murray 1987; Renkewitz and Sedlmeier 2007). Fisher (1890–1962), a British biologist, geneticist, and statistician, had only a null hypothesis in his theory of significance testing, but no alternative hypothesis. This null hypothesis could not be confirmed or supported by empirical data, but only be disproved: "...the null hypothesis is never proved or established, but is possibly disproved..."

(continued)

(Fisher 1935, p. 16). Neyman (1894–1981) and Pearson (1895–1980) extended Fisher's approach in that they explicitly introduced an alternative hypothesis and, like the null hypothesis, this alternative hypothesis was formulated in an exact way (e.g., Neyman and Pearson 1928). This also allows for a decision in favor of the null hypothesis, and we will return to related concepts such as the Type II error or power in Chap. 7. In addition, Neyman and Pearson interpreted the results of a significance test more cautiously, in that they did not encourage 'confirming' or 'rejecting' a hypothesis. Rather, they proposed a behavioral interpretation: One should *act* as if one hypothesis or the other were correct.

Fisher opposed the introduction of a H_1 (and its consequences) into his concept throughout his life, and this led to heated and personal disputes. For example, Fisher opened a discussion after a lecture by Jerzy Neyman at the Royal Statistical Society by saying that Neyman would have done better to choose a topic "on which he could speak with authority" (Neyman 1967, p. 193).

Difference Hypotheses for Up to Two Means: *t*-Tests

This chapter covers the *t*-test, one of the most widely used statistical tests. Strictly speaking, however, there is no such thing as "the" *t*-test; instead, we are looking at a family of statistical tests. The different versions tackle different study designs, and we distinguish three cases here: the *t*-test for independent samples (also called two-samples *t*-test), the *t*-test for dependent (or paired) samples, and the one-sample *t*-test. The first two variants assess whether an empirical difference in means is also indicative of differences in population means. The third variant compares a sample mean with an assumed population mean.

5.1 The *t*-Test for Two Independent Samples

Following our example from the previous chapters, we examine the substantive hypothesis *"More cigars are rolled in one hour in daylight than in artificial light."* First, we transform this (directional) hypothesis into its statistical formulation:

$$H_0 : \mu_{\text{daylight}} \leq \mu_{\text{artificial light}} \quad \text{and} \quad H_1 : \mu_{\text{daylight}} > \mu_{\text{artificial light}}$$

or, more generally.

$$H_0 : \mu_A \leq \mu_B \quad \text{and} \quad H_1 : \mu_A > \mu_B.$$

Our goal is to decide between these two hypotheses, and we will use the *t*-test for two independent samples to achieve this goal. In the simulation in Sect. 4.2 we had employed a simple scenario by assessing the probability of certain mean differences $D = M_A - M_B$, and Fig. 4.2 suggested that mean differences follow a normal distribution. Unfortunately,

© Springer-Verlag GmbH Germany, part of Springer Nature 2023
M. Janczyk, R. Pfister, *Understanding Inferential Statistics*,
https://doi.org/10.1007/978-3-662-66786-6_5

we usually do not know the parameters of this distribution, and we have to estimate, for example, the population variance from the data.

We now determine the expected value and variance of a random variable that assigns to each pair of two samples the difference of their means:

- Determining the *expected value* $E(M_A - M_B)$ is straightforward, because $E(M_A - M_B) = E(M_A) - E(M_B) = \mu_A - \mu_B$. Thus, the mean difference is an unbiased estimator for the difference between the population parameters μ_A and μ_B.
- Determining the *variance* $\sigma^2_{(M_A - M_B)}$ is a little more complicated unfortunately so that we only give the corresponding formula here (see Box 5.1 for details):

$$\sigma^2_{(M_A - M_B)} = \frac{(n_A - 1)\hat{S}_A^2 + (n_B - 1)\hat{S}_B^2}{n_A + n_B - 2} \left(\frac{1}{n_A} + \frac{1}{n_B} \right).$$

In Depth 5.1: The Variance of Differences of Means

To determine the variance for the difference between two means, we use the fact that the samples were drawn independently. Under this assumption we get:

$$\sigma^2_{(M_A - M_B)} = \sigma^2_{M_A} + \sigma^2_{M_B}.$$

We already know how to compute the variance of individual means (Formula 3.2): It is the variance of the population divided by the sample size. Now we assume that the variance is identical in both populations (see Sect. 5.1.4), which yields:

$$\sigma^2_{(M_A - M_B)} = \sigma^2_{M_A} + \sigma^2_{M_B} = \frac{\sigma^2}{n_A} + \frac{\sigma^2}{n_B} = \sigma^2 \left(\frac{1}{n_A} + \frac{1}{n_B} \right).$$

Finally, we estimate the population variance by weighting the individual (corrected) sample variances:

$$\hat{\sigma}^2 = \frac{(n_A - 1)\hat{S}_A^2 + (n_B - 1)\hat{S}_B^2}{n_A + n_B - 2}.$$

Taken together, the variance of the mean difference therefore is

$$\sigma^2_{(M_A - M_B)} = \frac{(n_A - 1)\hat{S}_A^2 + (n_B - 1)\hat{S}_B^2}{n_A + n_B - 2} \left(\frac{1}{n_A} + \frac{1}{n_B} \right).$$

In Chap. 3, we termed the root of a mean's variance the standard error of the mean. Similarly, we call the root of the variance, that is, $\sqrt{\sigma^2_{(M_A - M_B)}}$, the **standard error of the mean difference.** If we now compute the ratio of the mean difference and its standard error, we call the resulting ratio the **(empirical) *t*-ratio** or ***t*-value**

$$t = \frac{M_A - M_B}{\sqrt{\frac{(n_A-1)\hat{S}_A^2 + (n_B-1)\hat{S}_B^2}{n_A + n_B - 2}} \cdot \sqrt{\frac{1}{n_A} + \frac{1}{n_B}}}. \tag{5.1}$$

This general equation allows the two samples to be of different size. If the two samples are of the same size, we can simplify the equation to:

$$t = \frac{M_A - M_B}{\sqrt{\frac{\hat{S}_A^2 + \hat{S}_B^2}{n}}} \quad \text{with } n = n_A = n_B. \tag{5.2}$$

The *t*-value is an example of a so-called **test statistic**, and it has two important properties that we will re-encounter for all other test statistics:

- The absolute value of the ratio becomes larger the more the data speak against the H_0. This is especially evident for large differences between the empirical means, because this difference is in the numerator of the ratio.
- Similar to what we did in Sect. 4.2, we now assume that the H_0 is true, that is, we assume both samples to come from the same population. Let us now consider a continuous random variable *t* that assigns to each pair of two samples the corresponding *t*-value (i.e., the right part of Formula 5.1). Under this assumption. it is possible to determine the probability density function (or distribution) of such a random variable: The test statistic is *t*-distributed with $n_A + n_B - 2$ degrees of freedom. This fact can also be written as $t \overset{H_0}{\sim} t_{n_A + n_B - 2}$. Note that the *t*-distribution comes with several additional assumptions in addition to assuming the H_0 to be true (we will get back to this point in Sect. 5.1.4). We now discuss how a *t*-distribution looks like and what the term *degrees of freedom* means in this context.

5.1.1   The *t*-Distribution

Even if a variable can be assumed to follow a normal distribution in the population, corresponding test statistics actually require different distributions to accomodate measurement error. This is the case especially when working with small samples. William Gosset, a mathematician and chemist, routinely encountered these situations while working at the Guinness Brewery in Dublin. He published his foundational work on the *t*-distribution in

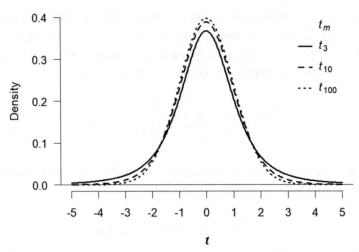

Fig. 5.1 Probability density functions of central t-distributions with different degrees of freedom m

1908, using the pseudonym of *Student*, because his employer had prohibited publication (Student 1908).

We focus on the so-called **central t-distribution** here. Like the normal distribution, this distribution is a whole family of possible t-distributions. The central t-distribution is symmetric around zero, but the exact shape depends on a parameter called the *degrees of freedom* of the distribution (abbreviated as *df*).[1] Figure 5.1 showcases three central t-distributions with different degrees of freedom m. The exact number of degrees of freedom depends mainly on the sample size. With large samples (and thus many degrees of freedom), the t-distribution approaches the standard normal distribution. If a random variable X follows a central t-distribution with m degrees of freedom (written as $X \sim t_m$), its expected value is $E(X) = 0$ (for $m > 1$) and its variance is $\sigma_X^2 = \frac{m}{m-2}$ (for $m > 2$).

5.1.2   Decisions Based on Critical t-Values

In the last two sections, we have learned about the test statistic t and its distribution. We now use these concepts to derive a simple rule for deciding between H_0 and H_1. This rule is a classic decision rule found in most textbooks on inferential statistics and it is routinely taught in corresponding courses. In the next section, we consider a variant of this rule that has become much more prevalent as a consequence of recent statistical developments and

---

[1] Later, we will also cover the non-central t-distribution, which plays an important role in the context of statistical power and Type II errors (see Chap. 7). Non-central distributions have an additional (non-zero) "non-centrality parameter".

the availability of statistical software. Both rules lead to the same decision, however (see also Sect. 4.2.3).

In Depth 5.2: What Are Degrees of Freedom?

The statistical concept of **degrees of freedom** has two different (and relatively abstract) meanings: One refers to empirical data, the other to parameters of probability density functions.

With respect to *empirical data*, the degrees of freedom indicate the number of elements of a data set which one can "freely choose". Initially, then, they are identical to the number of observations (usually n). However, degrees of freedom are "lost" if certain population parameters have to be estimated from the data in order to calculate further parameters. If, for example, we wanted to estimate the variance at the population level, we would have to calculate the mean value of the data first and use this value as an estimator for the population mean (cf. Sect. 3.4). By fixing the mean of the data, only $n - 1$ data points can be freely chosen. To illustrate this, consider a sample of size $n = 5$. Obviously, if nothing else is known about the sample, the five measured values can vary completely arbitrarily, and we cannot make any predictions about individual values. Thus, the degrees of freedom as the number of freely chosen elements are $df = 5$. However, if for some reason the mean of the sample is known, this is no longer true. For example, if we assume that the mean is $M = 10$, then we can only choose four values arbitrarily so that we can still find a fifth value to realize this particular mean, and this value therefore cannot be chosen freely anymore. For example, if we choose the values 8, 8, 12, and 12, it is clear that the fifth value must be exactly 10. Thus, the data in the sample are no longer completely arbitrary, and this is expressed by the loss of one degree of freedom ($df = 4$).

As *parameters of probability density functions*, degrees of freedom determine the exact shape of these functions (cf. Fig. 5.1). Thus, they (partially) compensate for the larger measurement inaccuracy when using small samples to estimate a population parameter. Like degrees of freedom for empirical data, they also depend on the size of the sample and a degree of freedom is lost whenever other distribution parameters (e.g., the mean) have to be estimated from the data in order to calculate certain parameters.

The family of *t*-tests discussed in this chapter illustrates this fact particularly clearly: For the *t*-test for independent samples, the two mean values of the samples are required to calculate the relevant standard error. This means that two degrees of freedom are lost. Accordingly, we use here a *t*-distribution with $n_A + n_B - 2$ degrees of freedom. For the one-sample *t*-test and the *t*-test for two dependent samples (see Sects. 5.2 and 5.3), we only need one mean to calculate the relevant standard error, and we therefore use a distribution with $n - 1$ degrees of freedom instead.

In Sect. 2.2.1 we had mentioned that for continuous random variables, single values do not have a particular probability (the probability of each of the infinitesimally many values is zero) so that actual probabilities can only be given for ranges of values. The probability of observing a value within this range is the area under the probability density function between the endpoints of this range. Furthermore, we had already mentioned that the total area under a probability density function from $-\infty$ to $+\infty$ is always 1.

Similarly, it is possible to find a value to the right of which (up to $+\infty$) there is a certain proportion of the area under the probability density function (see Box 2.3). We call this proportion of the area α and the value we are looking for is the **critical value** (see also Sect. 4.2.2). If we assume the probability density function to be a t-distribution, we would call this value the "critical t-value"—or t_{crit} for short. To determine t_{crit}, we use the following integral:

$$\int_{t_{\text{crit}}}^{\infty} f(x)dx = \alpha,$$

where $f(x)$ is the probability density function of the t-distribution. Fortunately, common statistics books provide tables of critical values for various degrees of freedom and specific values of α, so we do not need to solve integrals at this point.[2] Moreover, computer programs such as R allow us to quickly determine these critical values for many types of distributions (see Sect. 5.5). For $\alpha = 0.05$ and a t-distribution with ten degrees of freedom, this value is $t_{\text{crit}} = 1.81$. This case is illustrated in Fig. 5.2: The area shaded in gray accounts for exactly 5% of the total area under the probability density function. In other words: The probability of randomly drawing one particular value from a t-distributed random variable that is larger than or equal to t_{crit} is always less than or equal to α, thus: $P(t \geq t_{\text{crit}}) \leq \alpha$.

We already know that a random variable t, which assigns to any pair of two samples the empirical t-value (Formulas 5.1 and 5.2), is t-distributed with $n_A + n_B - 2$ degrees of freedom. As described above, this is only true if the two samples are drawn from the same population—that is, the H_0 is true—and if certain other preconditions are met (cf. Sect. 5.1.4). Conducting a study now corresponds to randomly drawing one value of this random variable. The probability of obtaining an empirical t-value that is larger than or equal to the critical t-value is always less than or equal to α. The logic of the decision is then completely analogous to the one we had introduced in Chap. 4: Larger (absolute) empirical t-values speak against H_0, and if our empirical t-value (or a larger one) is very unlikely if the H_0 is true, then we question this assumption and decide in favor of the H_1.

---

[2] Some tables provide the area from $-\infty$ up to the critical value instead. Thus, if working with $\alpha = 0.05$ (i.e., 5% of the total area should lie to the right of this value), we would have to look up the column for a proportion of $1 - 0.05 = 0.95$ (i.e., 95% of the total area should lie to the left of the critical value in this case).

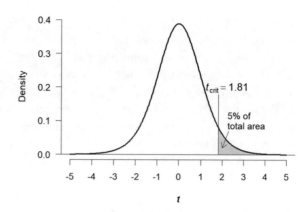

Fig. 5.2 Probability density function of a *t*-distribution with ten degrees of freedom: t_{crit} is the value to the right of which there is 5% of the total area (shaded gray). This area is called α. We thus have $\alpha = 0.05$

Let $t_{n_A+n_B-2;\alpha}$ be the critical *t*-value, to the right of which there is $\alpha \cdot 100\,\%$ of the area under the *t*-distribution with $n_A + n_B - 2$ degrees of freedom. Then, the decision rule is:

$$\text{Reject the } H_0, \text{ if } t \geq t_{n_A+n_B-2;\alpha}.$$

An important question is now (again): What do we want to call "very unlikely" (cf. Sect. 4.2.2)? The answer is: α. By convention, most studies use $\alpha = 0.05$ or $\alpha = 0.01$, and this α is what is called **significance level**. It therefore gives the probability with which the empirical (or a more extreme) *t*-value is allowed to occur without us questioning the assumption that the H_0 is true.

The central *t*-distribution does not, of course, preclude that large *t*-values may occur by chance despite the H_0 being true—this just happens very rarely. This possibility must be taken into account when interpreting any statistical test, but the described decision rule minimizes this error probability by choosing a relatively small α. We will come back to this in Chap. 7 in detail.

In Depth 5.3: Non-Significant Results

What do we actually mean when we say, "An experimental manipulation associated with the different levels of an independent variable has an effect on the dependent variable"? Implicitly, we are assuming that the different levels have no influence or effect on the dependent variable if the population means do not differ across those levels—indicated by a non-significant result. However, this also means that we must speak of *no influence* if the influence on the dependent variable is identical for all levels. We can therefore only detect influences of that *differ in strength*.

(continued)

For example, let us compare two samples that undergo two different diets. If a subsequent *t*-test for the comparison of both groups does not lead to a significant result, it is still possible that both diets were effective—just not to different degrees.

This illustrates how important it is to choose the levels of the independent variables wisely and, for example, to work with control groups that differ from the experimental groups only in the manipulation of interest while being identical in all other aspects.

5.1.3 Decisions Based on *p*-Values

The last section had introduced the conventional rule for deciding between the two hypotheses. This is the approach of choice if we calculate a *t*-test "by hand" and only have a statistics book with appropriate tables available.

There are good reasons to consider an alternative decision rule, however. This rule leads to the same decision, but has additional advantages and is therefore the preferred option in practice. It is also routinely used in journal articles, theses, and the like. Most tests today are calculated with statistical programs that include an exact *p*-value in their output. This value can, of course, be used to decide between the two hypotheses just as well. In fact, the widely used guidelines of the American Psychological Association (APA 2020) require reporting precisely that *p*-value (with three decimals).[3] This also allows readers to judge for themselves if a *p*-value is close to the decision threshold.

But what does this *p*-value actually indicate? In the discussion in the previous section, we had stated that the probability for $t \geq t_{crit}$ is equal to or smaller than α, but we did not consider the exact probability for an empirical *t*-value. To determine this, we would have to compute the area under the probability density function from t to $+\infty$—and the *p*-value is precisely this area (see Sect. 4.2.3):

$$p = \int_{t_{empirical}}^{\infty} f(x)dx,$$

if $f(x)$ is a probability density function of the *t*-distribution.

---

[3] Deviating from this, the German Psychological Society (Deutsche Gesellschaft für Psychologie, DGPs) recommends a precision of two decimals for statistical parameters, but advocates exclusively reporting effect sizes instead of *p*-values (DGPs 2007, pp. 34, 48). We will discuss the concept of an effect size in Chap. 7.

In sum, the value of p is the (conditional) probability of the observed data (or even more extreme data) when assuming H_0 to be true:

$$p = P(\text{data}|H_0). \tag{5.3}$$

Determining such an exact **p-value** in practice does not require any actual integral calculus by hand. In Sect. 5.5 we will discuss how computer programs can be used to determine an exact p-value for any empirical t-value. Fortunately, it does not matter whether we make a decision on the basis of a critical t-value or on the basis of the p-value. The decision is always the same and depends primarily on what information we have available. That is:

$$t_{\text{empirical}} \geq t_{\text{crit}} \Leftrightarrow p \leq \alpha.$$

In both cases, we speak of a **statistically significant result** and have "good reasons" to decide in favor of the H_1—because we have determined in advance (!) how large α is. However, if we do not have a significant result, we lack these good reasons, and we tentatively decide to continue assuming that the H_0 is true (for more information on this, see Chap. 7).

In Depth 5.4: A Note on the Interpretation of p

As Formula 5.3 states, p is the conditional probability of the data (or more extreme data) under the assumption that the H_0 is true. In Sect. 4.2.3 we have already seen that the converse statement for conditional probabilities does not hold. Therefore, p can never be interpreted as the probability of the hypotheses being true in light of the data. The p-value thus never indicates the probability of the null hypothesis being true, but instead it always indicates the probability of the observed (or more extreme) data if the H_0 were true in the population.

Occasionally, significant results (e.g., for $\alpha = 0.05$) are interpreted as if there was a probability of 0.95 (or 95%) for the samples to come from two different populations. This interpretation is incorrect, too, because both samples either come from two populations (in which case the probability is 1.0) or they do not (in which case it is 0.0). A correct interpretation is: Suppose that in the population the H_0 were true and we were to draw two samples of the same size from this population for infinitely many times and then calculate the empirical t-value. Then, in only 5% of these cases would the t-value be larger than t_{crit}. For any actual study with significant results, the researcher has to hope not to have one of these rare cases at hand and thus come to an erroneous decision.

5.1.4   Assumptions

We have claimed that the random variable t follows a t-distribution. However, this assertion rests on several assumptions. In case of the t-test for two independent samples there are three important assumptions (for details on the first two assumptions, see also Box 5.1):

- The samples must be *drawn randomly* and they have to be *independent* of one another. This must be ensured by an appropriate experimental design. (We will discuss the case of dependent samples in Sect. 5.3).
- The dependent variable must be *normally distributed* in the population. The expected values of the two populations may differ, but the variances must be identical—or assumed to be identical (often called *homogeneity of variance* or *homoscedasticity*). The latter can be tested, for example, with Levene's test (Levene 1960).
- Since mean values and variances are included in the calculations, the measured variable must meet the level of an *interval scale*—or at least this must be assumed.

If one (or more) of these assumptions is not met (or is not assumed to be met), then it is not possible to derive the exact distribution of the random variable t, and the t-test behaves "liberally": The probability of significant results exceeds α even if H_0 is true in the population. In other words, the test comes with an inflated probability of an erroneous decision for the H_1 (the Type I error).

Fortunately, the t-test is relatively robust to violations of these assumptions. For sample sizes of $n \geq 30$, violations of the normality assumption are not critical. Because of the *central limit theorem*, the sample means then distribute approximately normally, and this is the actual assumption to be met (Kubinger et al. 2009). Even moderate violations of the homogeneity of variance appear not to be detrimental to the robustness of the t-test (Kubinger et al. 2009; Rasch and Guiard 2004). For strong violations of this assumption, however, choosing Welch's test is often recommended (Welch 1947), which is a generalization of the t-test to the case of unequal variances. The t-value is calculated slightly differently in this case, because a weighted averaging of the two variances no longer makes sense:

$$t = \frac{M_A - M_B}{\sqrt{\frac{\hat{S}_A^2}{n_A} + \frac{\hat{S}_B^2}{n_B}}}.$$

In addition, the degrees of freedom used for the **Welch test** are adjusted as follows (often rounded down):

$$df_{\text{corr}} = \frac{1}{\frac{c^2}{n_A - 1} + \frac{(1-c)^2}{n_B - 1}} \qquad \text{with} \qquad c = \frac{\frac{\hat{S}_A^2}{n_A}}{\frac{\hat{S}_A^2}{n_A} + \frac{\hat{S}_B^2}{n_B}}.$$

Sometimes, appropriate transformations also help, for example, to achieve a normal distribution of the data. Another alternative, especially for data not meeting interval scale level, are so-called non-parametric procedures (in this case the Mann-Whitney U-test; see e.g. Bortz and Schuster 2010; Hollander et al. 2014).

5.1.5 Testing Non-directional Hypotheses

So far we have used the *t*-test only in the case of a directional $H_1 : \mu_A > \mu_B$. We are thus implicitly expecting larger mean values in sample A as compared to sample B, and the numerator of the *t*-ratio was deliberately defined as $M_A - M_B$ to obtain positive values for t in this case. Thus, particularly large *t*-values speak against the H_0.

For non-directional alternative hypotheses $H_1 : \mu_A \neq \mu_B$, there is no prediction about the direction of the postulated difference: the two parameters only differ in one way or another, and we also allow for the case $M_A < M_B$ (i.e., a potentially negative *t*-value). The decision rules we have encountered so far do not cover this case. The symmetry of the central *t*-distribution comes in handy here, though, and we could also decide in favor of the H_1 if we observe particularly large negative *t*-values—so there are effectively two critical *t*-values: t_{crit} and $-t_{\text{crit}}$. To keep the total area at α, we do not "cut off" the entire area on one side of the distribution, but we cut off $\frac{\alpha}{2}$ on both sides in this case. The decision rule is thus:

> Reject the H_0, if $t \geq t_{n_A + n_B - 2; \frac{\alpha}{2}}$ or if $t \leq -t_{n_A + n_B - 2; \frac{\alpha}{2}}$.

We can also work with the absolute value of t and then the decision rule simplifies to:

> Reject the H_0, if $|t| \geq t_{n_A + n_B - 2; \frac{\alpha}{2}}$.

When deciding based on exact p-values, we need to be particularly mindful on how to calculate p in the non-directional case. Just as with critical *t*-values, we now need to consider the area at the left *and* at the right end of the *t*-distribution. Taking into account the symmetry of *t*-distributions, p is calculated as:

$$p = \int_{-\infty}^{-|t|_{\text{empirical}}} f(x)dx + \int_{+|t|_{\text{empirical}}}^{+\infty} f(x)dx = 2 \cdot \int_{+|t|_{\text{empirical}}}^{+\infty} f(x)dx,$$

if $f(x)$ is a probability density function of the *t*-distribution.

In Depth 5.5: *t*-Tests with Computer Programs
When analyzing data with computer programs, it is not always obvious whether the *t*-test has been performed for a directional or a non-directional alternative hypothesis. By default, both SPSS and R perform two-sided tests, that is, they test for non-directional hypotheses. While R allows for specifying directional alternative hypotheses with the `alternative` option, the *p*-value in the output of SPSS has to be divided by two in this case.

5.1.6   An Exemplary Calculation

Before discussing further members of the family of *t*-tests, we showcase an exemplary calculation here by using the data from Sect. 3.1.1. Suppose that we had theoretical reasons to expect performance in cigar rolling to be better in daylight than in artificial light. Hence, we formulate a directional alternative hypothesis and want to test it with $\alpha = 0.05$:

$$H_0 : \mu_{\text{daylight}} \leq \mu_{\text{artificial light}} \quad \text{and} \quad H_1 : \mu_{\text{daylight}} > \mu_{\text{artificial light}}.$$

We had already calculated the means of both samples in Sect. 3.1.1 ($M_{\text{daylight}} = 21.7$ and $M_{\text{artificial light}} = 18.7$) and we now have to convert the sample variances calculated there into the corrected sample variances:

$$\hat{S}^2_{\text{daylight}} = \frac{n}{n-1} S^2_{\text{daylight}} = \frac{10}{9} \cdot 5.21 = 5.79$$

$$\hat{S}^2_{\text{artificial light}} = \frac{n}{n-1} S^2_{\text{artificial light}} = \frac{10}{9} \cdot 5.81 = 6.46.$$

Since both samples are of the same size, we can calculate the empirical *t*-value according to Formula 5.2:

$$t = \frac{M_A - M_B}{\sqrt{\frac{\hat{S}^2_A + \hat{S}^2_B}{n}}} = \frac{21.7 - 18.7}{\sqrt{\frac{5.79 + 6.46}{10}}} = 2.71.$$

As the critical value of the *t*-distribution with 18 degrees of freedom, we determine $t_{\text{crit}} = 1.73$. Alternatively, we can determine *p* exactly and obtain $p = 0.007$. Thus, we get $t \geq t_{\text{crit}}$ and $p \leq \alpha$, respectively, and we decide in favor of the alternative hypothesis.

5.2 The One-Sample *t*-Test

The one-sample *t*-test is used to test whether a given sample comes from a population with a known (or hypothesized) population mean. Intelligence tests, for example, are often calibrated to a population mean of 100, and a researcher might wonder whether the mean of their sample is significantly different from this population mean. In statistical terms, this would translate to $H_1 : \mu \neq 100$ and the corresponding null hypothesis would therefore be $H_0 : \mu = 100$.

The basic procedure for this *t*-test corresponds to that of the *t*-test for two independent samples, and the pair of hypotheses for a non-directional test is:

$$H_0 : \mu = \mu_0 \quad \text{and} \quad H_1 : \mu \neq \mu_0,$$

where μ_0 is the corresponding test value (in the example $\mu_0 = 100$). We can then plug the data from the sample into the formula to calculate an empirical *t*-value. The distribution of a random variable *t*, which assigns to each sample this *t*-value, can then be determined exactly—again assuming H_0 to be true. More precisely, the empirical *t*-value in the one-sample case is calculated as

$$t = \frac{M_X - \mu_0}{\frac{\hat{S}_X}{\sqrt{n}}}, \tag{5.4}$$

and the corresponding random variable is *t*-distributed with $n - 1$ degrees of freedom, that is, $t \overset{H_0}{\sim} t_{n-1}$. A decision between the two hypotheses is again made either by comparing the empirical *t*-value with a critical *t*-value or by comparing p with α:

> Reject the H_0, if $|t| \geq t_{n-1;\frac{\alpha}{2}}$ or if $p \leq \alpha$.

We have here used the case of a non-directional H_1; with a directional alternative hypothesis, we use α instead of $\frac{\alpha}{2}$.

As for the *t*-test for independent samples, the one-sample *t*-test assumes interval scale level and normal distribution of the dependent variable, as well as a randomly drawn sample. The corresponding non-parametric procedure is the Wilcoxon test (see, e.g., Bortz and Schuster 2010; Hollander et al. 2014).

5.3 The *t*-Test for Two Dependent Samples

A common case in experimental psychology and in intervention studies alike is that of **repeated measures:** One and the same sample provides data for several conditions. This implies that each value of one sample (or condition) directly maps onto a value of the second sample (or condition). In that case, we speak of **dependent samples** or **within-subject designs**. To illustrate this, consider the following two examples:

- *"Can more cigars be rolled per hour in daylight or in artificial light?"* We had previously operationalized this example as one group of participants rolling cigars in daylight and another group rolling cigars in artificial light—two independent samples. However, we could also perform a conceptually identical experiment by having each participant roll cigars once in daylight and once in artificial light. We would then have two values per participant and thus two dependent samples.
- *"Does coffee affect memory?"* This question could be investigated by having each participant work on a memory test (variable X_A), then drink three cups of black coffee, and again work on a memory test (variable X_B). Thus, there are again two measurements from each participant.

   More generally, of course, we could consider any kind of intervention here, not only drinking coffee, and the variables X_A and X_B can also be any other measure. A common additional example is the effectiveness of a clinical intervention (pretest X_A—intervention—posttest X_B).

Such situations can be evaluated with a *t*-test for dependent (or paired) samples. It is important to note that the general performance level of the participants (e.g., their memory or reaction time, etc.) is not of interest to us in this case. Rather, it is only the difference between the two conditions for each individual participant that matters. We will discuss advantages and disadvantages of such research designs in Sect. 10.3.

Conceptually, the *t*-test for two dependent samples is only a special case of the one-sample *t*-test, and we therefore do not need a new test statistic. In contrast to the *t*-test for two independent samples, now A and B in the hypotheses do not represent populations or samples of different individuals, but of two different conditions for which there is data from each participant in the sample. In the non-directional case, the pair of hypotheses is:

$$H_0 : \mu_A = \mu_B \quad \text{and} \quad H_1 : \mu_A \neq \mu_B.$$

However, we can also formulate this pair of hypotheses somewhat differently—but in a mathematically equivalent way—by considering the difference $\mu_A - \mu_B$:

$$H_0 : \mu_A - \mu_B = 0 \quad \text{and} \quad H_1 : \mu_A - \mu_B \neq 0.$$

In other words, if μ_A and μ_B do not differ, their difference is, of course, zero. This allows us to actually treat the case of two dependent samples with the one-sample *t*-test introduced above: We calculate a new variable $D = X_A - X_B$ (thus, for each participant, we calculate the difference of their value in conditions A and B), and then test this new variable D with a one-sample *t*-test against the parameter $\mu_0 = 0$.

5.4 Summary

The basic procedure of performing a t-test is identical across all three variants (and, strictly speaking, also for other significance tests). It can be summarized in four steps:

1. First, we construct a pair of hypotheses (if possible based on theoretical considerations). Usually, the alternative hypothesis H_1 describes the predicted difference in terms of population parameters. The H_0 describes the opposite, including the case of equal means. We then aim to decide between these hypotheses: We reject the H_0 (i.e., decide in favor of the H_1), if the empirical (or even more extreme) data are very unlikely when assuming H_0 to be true.
2. To define what "very unlikely" means, we specify the significance level α. The conventional choice in the scientific community is either $\alpha = 0.05$ or $\alpha = 0.01$—but there are also justified exceptions to these consensus values.
3. We draw one or two (in-)dependent random sample(s) and compute appropriate sample statistics from the data ($\bar{X}$, $\hat{S}_X^2$). From these, we calculate a test statistic; in the present case, the empirical t-value. Now we have two options:

   - We determine the critical t-value (which depends on α) and decide between the hypotheses by comparing the empirical and the critical t-value.
   - We determine the exact p-value and decide between the hypotheses by comparing the p-value with the pre-specified α.

4. The decision rule therefore is :

$$\boxed{\text{Reject the } H_0, \text{ if } t \geq t_{m;\alpha} \text{ or if } p \leq \alpha.}$$

In Depth 5.6: A t-Value is a t-Value is a t-Value

We have encountered two variants of the t-ratio in this chapter: One in the case of two independent samples (Formula 5.1) and one in the case of one sample or two dependent samples (Formula 5.4). Although both look different at first glance, they have the same structure. In general terms, a t-ratio is

$$t = \frac{T - \tau_0}{SE_T}, \tag{5.5}$$

where T is an estimator for a parameter τ, τ_0 is the assumed value of the parameter τ, and SE_T is the (estimated) standard error of T. In the case of the one-sample t-test, the numerator of the ratio consists of M_X as the estimator of the parameter of

(continued)

interest μ and a test value μ_0. The denominator is the (estimated) standard error of the mean. In the two-sample case, a mean difference is estimated with $(M_A - M_B)$, and the test value is usually $\tau_0 = 0$ (and is therefore omitted). The denominator is the standard error of the mean difference. We will encounter the *t*-ratio later again, and we should keep in mind its general form according to Formula 5.5.

5.5   Examples and Exercises

In the following, we will demonstrate how to compute the different *t*-tests with R and SPSS. The story behind the following examples may seem rather artificial at first glance— but in fact it was exactly this problem that led to the development of the *t*-test.[4]

5.5.1   *t*-Tests with R

- **Example 1:** Table 5.1 summarizes the average crop yield of two different barley fields from two different regions owned by the Guinness Brewery (the data are provided in the file 5_1_data_barley_fields.dat). The aim is to test whether the yields of the two areas differ significantly from each other ($\alpha = 0.05$). Since no further information is available about the two areas, we will use a non-directional alternative hypothesis.

    For the calculation with R, we assume that the data from Table 5.1 and the variables of the resulting data frame have been made available with the function attach(). The variable area encodes the area in question (the independent variable), and the variable yield encodes the corresponding yield (the dependent variable).

```
area
1 1 1 1 1 1 1 1 1 1 2 2 2 2 2 2 2 2 2 2

yield
41 29 44 35 27 32 33 36 36 39 20 25 21
34 25 39 27 24 23 31
```

---

[4] For additional information on the historical roots of the *t*-test, see the Wikipedia entry on its inventor William Sealy Gosset (http://en.wikipedia.org/wiki/William_Sealy_Gosset).

Area	Yield									
1	41	29	44	35	27	32	33	36	36	39
2	20	25	21	34	25	39	27	24	23	31

Table 5.1 Example data. Crop yield (in arbitrary units) for two barley fields

First, we use the Levene test to test whether homogeneity of variance can be assumed. This is done with the function `leveneTest()` from the package `car`:

```
library(car)            # load package
leveneTest(yield, area, center = "mean")

Levene's Test for Homogeneity of Variance...
                                    ...(center = "mean")
      Df  F value  Pr(>F)
group  1   0.2129    0.65
```

The output shows that the Levene test is not significant, $p = .650$, so we assume homogeneity of variance and specify this for the subsequent t-test. The t-test for independent samples can be performed by providing the function `t.test()` with the crop yields of area 1 as the first vector (x) and the yields of area 2 as the second vector (y). In addition, we specify that a non-directional H_1 should be tested and that we assume homogeneity of variance:

```
t.test(x = yield[area == 1],
       y = yield[area == 2],
       alternative = "two.sided",
       var.equal = TRUE)
```

The output clearly shows that the yields of the two areas are significantly different, $t(18) = 3.29$, $p = .004$. The same result is obtained by performing the test manually, as described in the online material. In addition (not shown here), the means for both groups and a confidence interval around their difference are provided in the output (see Chap. 6).

```
Two Sample t-test

data:  yield[area == 1] and
       yield[area == 2]
t = 3.2851, df = 18, p-value = 0.004114
alternative hypothesis: true difference
          in means is not equal to 0
```

Table 5.2 Example data.
Crop yield (in arbitrary units)
for 2 years

	Field									
Time	1	2	3	4	5	6	7	8	9	10
Yield 2012	20	25	21	34	25	39	27	24	23	31
Yield 2013	25	22	26	33	27	39	34	27	24	35

A simple and direct access to the results of the function is also provided by the function
t_out() of the package schoRsch. This function formats the results according
to APA specifications and also provides an appropriate measure of effect size (see
Chap. 7):

```
library(schoRsch)
t_out( t.test(...) )
```

```
Two Sample t-test: t(18) = 3.29, p =.004, d = 1.47
```

- **Example 2:** A new fertilizer is introduced on the less productive fields from the first
  example to increase yields (Table 5.2; provided in the file 5_2_data_fertilizer.
  dat).

     Does this procedure actually increase yield? As in Example 1, we assume that
  the data from both measurement dates are available as variables (yield_2012 and
  yield_2013). The *t*-test for dependent samples is also called via the function
  t.test(). In addition, a directed alternative hypothesis is now appropriate; those
  data are taken as argument x, for which the larger mean is expected:

```
t.test(x = yield_2013,
       y = yield_2012,
       alternative = "greater",
       paired = TRUE)
```

The output shows that the empirical increase in yield is statistically significant, $t(9) =$
$2.35, p = .022$.

```
Paired t-test

data:  yield_2013 and yield_2012
t = 2.3515, df = 9, p-value = 0.0216
alternative hypothesis: true difference
    in means is greater than 0
```

Formatting via the function t_out() is possible as well:

```
Paired t-test: t(9) = 2.35, p =.022, d = 1.05
```

- **Example 3:** A Guinness clerk wants to re-examine the change from Example 2, but only has access to the change in yield (i.e., the difference in yield between the two harvests for each field). In this case, the analysis can still be performed by testing the mean difference against the value of 0 using a one-sample *t*-test. Thus, we first compute the differences from the two existing variables:

```
fertilizer_effect <- yield_2013 - yield_2012
```

The data of the new variable `fertilizer_effect` can then be tested against the value $\mu_0 = 0$ with the function `t.test()`. No second data vector is specified because this is a one-sample *t*-test:

```
t.test(x = fertilizer_effect,
       alternative = "greater",
       mu = 0)
```

The output is the same as in Example 2.

In addition, R offers convenient ways to directly access distributions and query specific values. We here use the example of the *t*-distribution to demonstrate this.

- **Example 4:** We are looking for the value that cuts off 5% of the area of a *t*-distribution with eleven degrees of freedom, whereby the 5% are to be divided equally between both tails of the distribution. This example also shows how to calculate a critical *t*-value.

    With R, we determine those values of the *t*-distribution that cut off 2.5% of the area to the left and right, respectively. This can be done with the function `qt()` ("quantiles of the *t*-distribution"), which requires as arguments (1) the area to be cut from the left and (2) the degrees of freedom of the *t*-distribution:

```
qt(0.975,11) # 97.5% from -infinity
qt(0.025,11) #  2.5% from -infinity


 2.200985
-2.200985
```

- **Example 5:** A researcher has calculated an empirical *t*-value of 2.54. The task is to determine how likely such a value or a more extreme value is, assuming a *t*-distributed test statistic with 15 degrees of freedom?

    First, the function `pt()` can be used to determine the area which is cut off by any *t*-value from a given distribution. The area is always determined from $-\infty$ up to the specified *t*-value. The difference of this value to 1 therefore is the probability that we are looking for and it corresponds to the *p*-value of a one-sided *t*-test:

```
1-pt(2.54, 15)


0.01132112    # the test would be significant at alpha = 0.05.
```

5.5.2 *t*-Tests with SPSS

- **Example 1:** Table 5.3 summarizes the average crop yield of different barley fields from two large growing areas owned by the Guinness brewery (the data are provided in the file `5_1_data_barley_fields.sav`). The aim is to test whether the yields of the two areas differ significantly from each other ($\alpha = 0.05$). We test a non-directional alternative hypothesis, since we do not have any further information about the two areas.

  The SPSS file contains two variables (columns). The variable `Area` codes the two areas as 1 or 2, and the variable `Yield` provides the crop yield. To perform the *t*-test for independent samples, we open the menu

```
Analyze > Compare Means > Independent-Samples T Test...
```

  There we add the independent variable `Area` to the field *Grouping Variable*. The groups are then defined via *Define Groups...* by specifying the coding of the groups (1 or 2 in this example).

  We then add the variable `Yield` to the field *Test Variable(s)*. Clicking on *OK* starts the calculation and triggers the corresponding output (see Fig. 5.3). After the output of descriptive statistics for both groups, we find the inferential statistics in the second table. Columns 2 and 3 show the results of the Levene test. In our example, the test is not significant, $p = 0.650$, that is, we assume homogeneity of variance and consider

Table 5.3 Example data. Crop yield (in arbitrary units) of two fields

Area	Yield									
1	41	29	44	35	27	32	33	36	36	39
2	20	25	21	34	25	39	27	24	23	31

Group Statistics

	Area	N	Mean	Std. Deviation	Std. Error Mean
Yield	1	10	35.20	5.245	1.659
	2	10	26.90	6.027	1.906

Independent Samples Test

		Levene's Test for Equality of Variances		t-test for Equality of Means				
		F	Sig.	t	df	Sig. (2-tailed)	Mean Difference	Std. Error Difference
Yield	Equal variances assumed	.213	.650	3.285	18	.004	8.300	2.527
	Equal variances not assumed			3.285	17.663	.004	8.300	2.527

Fig. 5.3 SPSS output for a *t*-test for independent samples

Table 5.4 Example data. Crop yield (in arbitrary units) for 2 years

Time	Field 1	2	3	4	5	6	7	8	9	10
Yield 2012	20	25	21	34	25	39	27	24	23	31
Yield 2013	25	22	26	33	27	39	34	27	24	35

Paired Samples Statistics

		Mean	N	Std. Deviation	Std. Error Mean
Pair 1	Yield_2013	29.20	10	5.613	1.775
	Yield_2012	26.90	10	6.027	1.906

Paired Samples Correlations

		N	n	Sig.
Pair 1	Yield_2013 & Yield_2012	10	.861	.001

Paired Samples Test

		Paired Differences Mean	Std. Deviation	Std. Error Mean	t	df	Sig. (2-tailed)
Pair 1	Yield_2013 - Yield_2012	2.300	3.093	.978	2.352	9	.043

Fig. 5.4 SPSS output for a *t*-test for dependent samples

the upper row *(Equal variances assumed)* in the following table. There, we can find values such as the empirical *t*-value *(t)*, the degrees of freedom *(df)*, and the *p*-value *(Sig. 2-tailed)*. The *t*-test is thus significant, $t(18) = 3.29$, $p = .004$.

- **Example 2:** A new fertilizer is introduced on the less productive fields from the first example to increase yields (Table 5.4; these data are provided in the file 5_2_data_fertilizer.sav). Does this procedure actually increase the yield significantly?

  In this case, for SPSS, the data must be provided as two variables (Yield_2012 and Yield_2013). In order to use the *t*-test for dependent samples, we open the menu

```
Analyze > Compare Means > Paired-Samples T Test...
```

There, we select the two variables to be compared in the left list. Clicking on *OK* opens the output (Fig. 5.4). Again, descriptive statistics are provided in the first table, while the correlation of both variables is reported in the second table (cf. Chap. 11). The third table then contains the inferential statistical results, such as the empirical *t*-value, the degrees of freedom, and the *p*-value. The output $p = .043$, however, is calculated in

SPSS for a non-directional H_1. Since we have a directional hypothesis in this case, we need to divide this value by 2, $t(9) = 2.35$, $p = .022$.

- **Example 3:** A Guinness clerk wants to re-examine the change from Example 2, but only has access to the change in yield (i.e., the difference in yields between the two harvests for each field). In this case, the test can still be performed by testing the mean difference against zero using a one-sample *t*-test. First, we calculate the differences from the two existing variables. To do this, we select the menu

```
Transform > Compute Variable...
```

and enter the desired name of the new variable (Fertilizer Effect) in the field *Target Variable*. Further, we specify the calculation in the field *Numeric Expression*, in this case yield_2013-yield_2012. This new variable can now be tested against 0 with the one-sample *t*-test:

```
Analyze > Compare Means > One-Sample T-Test...
```

In the field *Test Value*, we specify the value against which the mean of the selected variable should be tested. By default, this value is already set to 0. The result (Fig. 5.5) is the same as in Example 2. Again, note that tests in SPSS are usually for non-directional alternative hypotheses (i.e., two-sided) and that the *p*-value needs to be divided by 2 accordingly.

Unfortunately, direct access to distributions is not as easy with SPSS as it is with R (see Examples 4 and 5 in Sect. 5.5.1). Of course, this is no obstacle for the automated calculation of *t*-tests. Sometimes this information comes in handy, though, for instance,

One-Sample Statistics

	N	Mean	Std. Deviation	Std. Error Mean
FertilizerEffect	10	2.3000	3.09300	.97809

One-Sample Test

Test Value = 0

	t	df	Sig. (2-tailed)	Mean Difference
FertilizerEffect	2.352	9	.043	2.30000

Fig. 5.5 SPSS output for a one-sample *t*-test

when computing confidence intervals (see Chap. 6). A solution to this problem is possible by using common software such as MS Excel or Libre Office Calc (and the corresponding functions `T.DIST` and `T.INV`). Alternatively, numerous additional options with similar functions can be found on the internet (e.g., https://stattrek.com/online-calculator/t-distribution).

Confidence Intervals

6

We have seen in Chap. 3 how the population mean μ and the associated population variance σ^2 can be estimated with sample statistics. These estimators are usually referred to as **point estimators**. However, we can also go a step further and learn something about the precision of these estimates or calculate an interval that covers a range of plausible population parameters. This procedure is called **interval estimation** and the calculated intervals are known as **confidence intervals**. Confidence intervals are often used as error bars in figures, where they are intended to facilitate interpretation, because they allow to visually detect significant differences between values.

Although confidence intervals can theoretically be calculated for many different parameters, in practice this is most often done for the parameter μ. We will therefore focus on this case, starting with the general form of a confidence interval and then applying it to the (common) confidence interval for single sample means. We then contrast the concepts of null hypothesis significance testing and confidence intervals, and finally consider confidence intervals for dependent (paired) samples.

6.1 The General Form of Confidence Intervals

Confidence intervals describe an interval around a fixed value. This interval is usually symmetric, that is, of the same size to both sides of the fixed value. The entire range of an interval is called its width. If T is a fixed value and E is half the width of the interval, then the usual notation is

$$[T - E, T + E], \text{ or for short } [T \pm E].$$

© Springer-Verlag GmbH Germany, part of Springer Nature 2023
M. Janczyk, R. Pfister, *Understanding Inferential Statistics*,
https://doi.org/10.1007/978-3-662-66786-6_6

Each confidence interval consists of three elements and has the following form:

$$[T - c \cdot SE_T, T + c \cdot SE_T] \quad \text{or} \quad [T \pm c \cdot SE_T]. \tag{6.1}$$

Here, T denotes a suitable estimator for the population parameter of interest, for example, M when calculating a confidence interval for μ. SE_T is the standard error of T; the remaining parameter c is the "certainty parameter" which depends on the distribution of T and the intended precision of the confidence interval. In summary, then, any confidence interval can be reduced to the form "estimator $\pm$ certainty parameter $\cdot$ standard error of the estimator".

6.2   Confidence Intervals for Means

We now specify the general form of a confidence interval according to Formula 6.1 for a confidence interval of the parameter μ. Here we start directly with the common case that the population variance σ^2 is unknown and must therefore be estimated. This setting corresponds to that of a t-test (Chap. 5).

6.2.1   Calculation

Sample means follow a normal distribution, and we also know the two parameters of the corresponding distribution (cf. Formula 3.3):

$$\bar{X} \sim N\left(\mu, \frac{\sigma^2}{n}\right).$$

The square root of the variance of this random variable is the standard error of the mean (SE_M). Thus, we already know almost all components of the confidence interval we are looking for—apart from the certainty parameter c. At first glance, it seems obvious that this parameter is taken from the normal distribution. This would indeed be the case if we knew the population variance. However, because this is usually not the case, we have to estimate the population variance instead:

$$SE_M = \frac{\hat{S}_X}{\sqrt{n}}.$$

As a consequence, the means are no longer normally distributed, but follow a t-distribution—from which the certainty parameter c is determined. Since confidence intervals are usually calculated in a two-sided form,

$$\left[M_X \pm t_{n-1;\frac{\alpha}{2}} \cdot \frac{\hat{S}_X}{\sqrt{n}} \right] \tag{6.2}$$

is the $(1 - \alpha) \cdot 100\%$ confidence interval for μ. Here $t_{n-1;\frac{\alpha}{2}}$ is the t-value, to the left of which there is $(1 - \frac{\alpha}{2}) \cdot 100\%$ of the area of a t-distribution with $n - 1$ degrees of freedom.

6.2.2 Factors Influencing the Width of Confidence Intervals

Determining the center of a confidence interval is relatively easy: it is given by T, that is, the estimator of the parameter for which we calculate a confidence interval. The width of a confidence interval depends on three separate factors, however. Figure 6.1 illustrates this point by showcasing different confidence intervals.

6.2.3 Interpreting Confidence Intervals

What exactly does a confidence interval mean? One common interpretation—and a seemingly intuitive one—refers to the probability that the estimated population parameter lies within the confidence interval: Thus, with 95% probability, a population parameter should lie within the calculated 95% confidence interval (Rasch et al. 2010; see also Cousineau 2017; Cumming and Finch 2005).

It should be remembered, however, that the confidence or certainty of 95% is not a property of the population parameter: Indeed, the true population parameter either lies in the interval (in which case we have $p = 1.0$), or it does not lie in the interval (then is $p = 0.0$). Instead, it is a property of the estimation procedure and refers to how often a calculated confidence interval will actually include the population parameter. A correct interpretation is that if we were to repeatedly draw samples of size n from a population (for infinitely many times), then the population parameter would lie within the 95% confidence intervals in 95% of the repetitions. We have already encountered a similar interpretation in the field of hypothesis testing in Sect. 5.1.3.

Instead of a formal presentation, we illustrate this interpretation with a simulation (Fig. 6.2). This example is based on a normally distributed variable with an expected value $\mu = 50$ and a variance $\sigma^2 = 20$. We then drew 50 independent samples of size $n = 20$ from this population and for each sample, we calculated the 95% confidence interval according to Formula 6.2 and plotted the result. If an infinite number of such

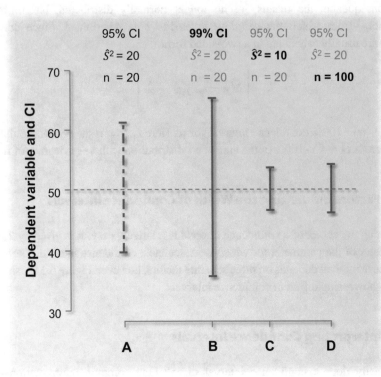

Fig. 6.1 Four different confidence intervals (CIs) of varying width; all confidence intervals are based on a sample that was drawn from a normally distributed population with $\mu = 50$. Since the population parameter is known in this example, all intervals are displayed as centered around this value. Confidence interval A serves as a baseline for comparisons, and confidence intervals B-D were computed by changing one of the three relevant variables each. For confidence interval B, this concerns the certainty parameter: Aiming for higher certainty (99% instead of 95%) leads to a wider confidence interval. Confidence interval C is based on a population with smaller variance. Since samples then tend to also have a smaller variance, this reduces the width of the interval. The same applies to confidence interval D, which is based on a larger sample, what generally reduces the standard error

samples had been drawn, one would expect 95% of the confidence intervals to include the true parameter $\mu = 50$. Thus, in the case of 50 samples, this should be true for about 47.5 of the 50 confidence intervals. In Fig. 6.2, solid lines indicate those confidence intervals that do *not* include the true parameter. In line with the above interpretation, the parameter is included in 47 of the 50 confidence intervals.

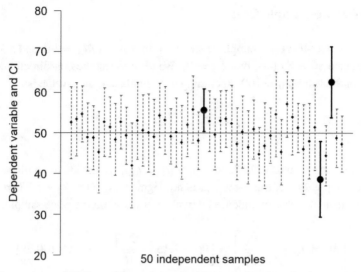

Fig. 6.2 Comparison of 95% confidence intervals (CIs) calculated on the basis of 50 randomly drawn samples from the same normally distributed population. The horizontal line indicates the true parameter $\mu = 50$ and the solid lines represent the confidence intervals that do not contain the parameter

6.3   Confidence Intervals and Hypothesis Testing

So far, we have treated confidence intervals and hypothesis testing as separate topics. Comparing the structure of a confidence interval for the parameter μ (Formula 6.2) and the t-value in the one-sample case (Formula 5.4) reveals several notable similarities, however:

$$\left[M_X \pm t_{n-1;\frac{\alpha}{2}} \cdot \frac{\hat{S}_X}{\sqrt{n}} \right] \quad \text{and} \quad t = \frac{M_X - \mu_0}{\frac{\hat{S}_X}{\sqrt{n}}} \overset{H_0}{\sim} t_{n-1}.$$

For example, the mean value M_X and the standard error of the mean $SE_M = \frac{\hat{S}_X}{\sqrt{n}}$ occur in both formulas. Moreover, both draw on the t-distribution with $n-1$ degrees of freedom. These similarities suggest a relationship between confidence intervals and significance tests, and both approaches indeed yield identical conclusions. However, confidence intervals provide additional information about the range of plausible values for the parameter and therefore about the precision of the estimate. The similarities are illustrated below with two examples.

6.3.1   The One-Sample Case

We first perform a t-test for a sample of size $n = 16$, a mean $M_X = 96$, and a (corrected) sample variance $\hat{S}_X^2 = 81$ (and thus $\hat{S}_X = 9$). We want to test the non-directional H_0 with $\alpha = 0.05$ for the value $\mu_0 = 100$. According to Formula 5.4, the t-value is:

$$t = \frac{96 - 100}{\frac{9}{\sqrt{16}}} = -1.\bar{7}.$$

The critical t-value would be 2.13, and since $|t| < t_{\text{crit}}$, we decide to continue assuming that the null hypothesis is true—the test is not significant, $t(15) = -1.78$, $p = 0.096$. Now we calculate the 95% confidence interval for μ based on the same sample:

$$\left[M_X \pm t_{n-1;\frac{\alpha}{2}} \cdot \frac{\hat{S}_X}{\sqrt{n}} \right] = \left[96 \pm 2.13 \cdot \frac{9}{\sqrt{16}} \right] = [91.21, 100.79].$$

Obviously, the test value $\mu_0 = 100$ is included in the 95% confidence interval around M_X. Indeed, this can be generalized: If μ_0 is included in the corresponding confidence interval, the one-sample t-test will not be significant. Or, the other way a round, if μ_0 is not included in the confidence interval, the one-sample t-test is significant.

6.3.2   Confidence Intervals for Differences Between Means

In Sect. 5.1 we introduced the t-test for two independent samples. Here we had a difference in means as the numerator of the corresponding t-ratio (see Formulas 5.1 and 5.2). We now want to calculate a confidence interval for the difference in means instead of the t-test. In fact, we already have all the information at hand that we need to specify the confidence interval based on its general form (Formula 6.1). First, the parameter we are looking for, that is, the difference $\mu_A - \mu_B$, can be estimated with the difference of the means of both samples, that is, with $M_A - M_B$. The certainty parameter is obtained from the t-distribution and thus is $t_{n_A + n_B - 2; \frac{\alpha}{2}}$. The last remaining piece is the standard error SE_T of the estimator. In Box 5.6 we already mentioned that the t-ratio has an estimator in the numerator and its standard error in the denominator—which is exactly what we are looking for.

We consider here two samples of the (same) size $n = 10$. Let the calculated means be $M_A = 55.5$ and $M_B = 71.0$ and the (corrected) sample variances be $\hat{S}_A^2 = 285.17$ and $\hat{S}_B^2 = 212.0$. Furthermore, we assume homogeneity of variance and a two-sided (non-directional) test with $\alpha = 0.05$. Plugging these values into Formula 5.2, we get $t = -2.20$.

The critical t-value would be 2.10. Because $|t| \geq t_{\text{crit}}$, the t-test is significant, and we reject the H_0 and assume that the H_1 is true instead. To calculate the 95% confidence interval for the difference between the means, we plug the appropriate values into Formula 6.1. Because of the identical sample sizes, we directly take the denominator from Formula 5.2 to estimate the standard error (in general, the denominator from Formula 5.1 is used for this purpose):

$$[T \pm c \cdot SE_T] = \left[(M_A - M_B) \pm t_{n_A + n_B - 2; \frac{\alpha}{2}} \cdot \sqrt{\frac{\hat{S}_A^2 + \hat{S}_B^2}{n}} \right]$$

$$= \left[-15.5 \pm 2.10 \cdot \sqrt{\frac{285.17 + 212.0}{10}} \right] \tag{6.3}$$

$$= [-30.31, -0.69].$$

The interpretation is similar to the one-sample case described above: If the test value (in this case a difference of zero) lies within the confidence interval, a t-test will not be significant. In our example, this is not the case—and the t-test is significant just as well, $t(18) = -2.20$, $p = 0.021$.

Note, however, that figures for two samples sometimes show confidence intervals for individual means rather than confidence intervals for differences. We revisit this issue in Sect. 6.5.

6.4   Confidence Intervals for Dependent Samples

In Sect. 5.3, we already discussed that dependent samples require a different approach than independent samples do. We further mentioned that differences in the overall level of performance across participants are usually not of interest when working with dependent samples. What is important instead, is how the two conditions differ within individual participants.

This peculiarity of dependent samples is just as important when calculating confidence intervals, which are often called "within-subject confidence intervals" (Cousineau 2005; Pfister and Janczyk 2013). Analogous to the t-test for dependent samples, we do not consider the measured values themselves, but their difference D, which is calculated for each element of the sample as $D = X_A - X_B$. The standard deviation of these differences tells us something about the consistency of the differences among all participants:

It becomes smaller the more similar the differences are. The standard error of these differences[1] is calculated as:

$$SE_D = \frac{\hat{S}_D}{\sqrt{n}}.$$

This enables us to calculate the $(1 - \alpha) \cdot 100\%$ confidence interval for dependent samples as:

$$\left[M_X \pm t_{n-1; \frac{\alpha}{2}} \cdot \frac{\hat{S}_D}{\sqrt{n}} \right]. \tag{6.4}$$

On closer inspection, this confidence interval has two important differences from the confidence interval for a mean (see Sect. 6.3.1):

- The confidence interval calculated in this way is the same for both means; the within-subject standard error cannot be calculated separately for each mean, as is possible with confidence intervals for independent samples.
- Centering this confidence interval around the two means allows for drawing conclusions about the difference between the means. In this case, a t-test for dependent samples is significant if, and only if, one mean is not within the confidence interval around the other mean. However, this confidence interval does not say anything about whether one of the two means is different from any fixed value (e.g., 0). In this respect, the interpretation of the within-subject confidence interval is analogous to the confidence interval for the difference between means for two independent samples (see Sect. 6.3.2).

6.5   Comparison of the Different Confidence Intervals

We will revisit the different types of confidence intervals discussed in this chapter and focus on what can be concluded from their graphical representation with regard to the difference between the (two) means (see also Pfister and Janczyk 2013). Even among empirical researchers, this issue often leads to striking misconceptions (Belia et al. 2005), whereas getting a firm grasp on this technique allows for efficient graphical communication of scientific results.

---

[1] Some alternative methods for computing confidence intervals for within-subject designs produce a width that is shorter by a factor of $\frac{1}{\sqrt{2}}$, but require a multiplication with $\sqrt{2}$ to assess whether pairwise differences are significant. This factor stems from the fact that another quantity can be used to calculate the standard error as well (Loftus and Masson 1994). However, this quantity requires additional concepts that we will introduce in the context of Analysis of variance and will therefore discuss this point in Chaps. 8 and 10.

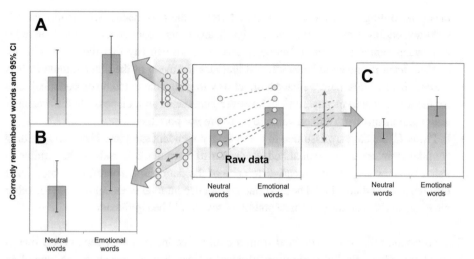

Fig. 6.3 Illustration of the confidence intervals discussed in this chapter. In Panels A and B, the raw data are assumed to come from two independent samples; in Panel C, they are assumed to come from dependent samples. In all cases, the error bars are 95% confidence intervals. In Panel A, these refer to the individual means, in Panels B and C to the difference in means

The following considerations refer to Fig. 6.3. The central panel of this figure shows five data points for two conditions (neutral vs. emotional words), that is, the number of words recalled in each condition. In all panels, the bars correspond to the means and the error bars are 95% confidence intervals. In Panels A and B, we assume that the data come from two independent samples, and in Panel C, we assume them to come from dependent samples (in the panel of the raw data, this is represented by the dashed lines connecting pairs of data points).

- **Panel A** shows confidence intervals for each of the two samples using Formula 6.2. Because the variance of both samples is different, the resulting confidence intervals also differ in width. What can be concluded from this graphical representation? First, both confidence intervals obviously do not include zero; thus, both means are significantly different from zero for $\alpha = 0.05$ (this corresponds to the one-sample t-test). Furthermore, the confidence interval on the right-hand side does not include the mean on the left-hand side. Does this mean that a t-test for two independent samples with $\alpha = 0.05$ would be significant? No—while this may be the case, it need not be true (in our example it is actually not the case, $p = .06$). A rule of thumb holds that a significant difference can be assumed if both confidence intervals overlap by no more than half of the average confidence interval. However, this is only true if certain conditions are met (e.g., sufficiently large samples and homogeneity of variance; see Cumming and Finch 2005).
- The confidence intervals in **Panel B** are both the same size, but they are also larger than those in Panel A: They correspond to the confidence interval for the difference between

means according to Formula 6.3, centered around the two means. We mentioned that a corresponding t-test would not be significant if this confidence interval includes zero when centered on the difference. Likewise, we can say that the t-test will not be significant if one confidence interval includes the mean of the other sample (this is the case here). Thus, here we have a direct way to gauge the outcome of statistical tests for the difference in means. In turn, however, statements about a possible difference of individual means from a fixed value (e.g., 0) are *not* possible.

- In **Panel C**, the data are assumed to come from dependent samples. The corresponding confidence intervals are calculated according to Formula 6.4, and—quite similar to Panel B—they refer to the mean difference of the data pairs. Therefore, a significant difference can be concluded here: If one confidence interval does not include the other mean (as in the example), a corresponding t-test would be significant.

The information that can be derived from a confidence interval thus depends on how it is calculated. This aspect also requires sufficiently clear descriptions about the type of an error bar in figure captions. For example, standard deviations do not tend to carry any meaningful information in the context of a figure, and standard errors and confidence intervals call for fundamentally different interpretations. More information on this can be found, for example, in Cousineau (2017), Cumming and Finch (2005), Dracup (2005), and Pfister and Janczyk (2013).

6.6   Confidence Intervals with R and SPSS

R and SPSS provide simple confidence intervals in their output by default when calculating, for example, a t-test (see Chap. 5). If two means are included in the t-test, then the confidence interval will automatically be computed for their difference. In the case of R, a two-sided test should also always be selected in order to obtain symmetrical confidence intervals. This confidence interval is often the more interesting one in practice, but a calculation of separate confidence intervals is of course also possible and is described briefly here.

To manually calculate a confidence interval with R, we first determine the critical quantile using the qt() function (see Example 4 in Sect. 5.5.1) and then multiply it with the standard error. The first argument passed to the qt() function is the desired "precision" as $1 - \frac{\alpha}{2}$ followed by the degrees of freedom. For a 95% confidence interval, the quantile is thus generated with the command qt(0.975, df). The relevant standard error is calculated in the same way as for the corresponding t-test (see also the online material for this example).[2]

---

[2] Options for calculating confidence intervals are also provided by the R package Rmisc.

| | | | t-test for Equality of Means | |
| | | | 95% Confidence Interval of the Difference | |
Sig. (2-tailed)	Mean Difference	Std. Error Difference	Lower	Upper
.004	8.300	2.527	2.992	13.608
.004	8.300	2.527	2.985	13.615

Fig. 6.4 Part of an SPSS output for a *t*-test for independent samples using the data from Table 5.3. The two right columns show lower and upper bounds of the 95% confidence interval around the mean difference

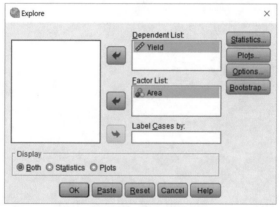

Fig. 6.5 *Exploratory data analysis* dialog box in SPSS. This function provides, among other things, confidence intervals for sample means

Figure 6.4 shows the relevant parts of the output when calculating a *t*-test (for two independent samples) with SPSS: The last two columns contain the lower and upper bounds, respectively, of the confidence interval around the difference (in Fig. 5.4 we had cut these two columns from the corresponding table).

To calculate confidence intervals manually with SPSS, we can also use the menu

`Analyze > Descriptive Statistics > Explore...`

In the dialog box (Fig. 6.5), we enter the dependent variable(s) in the field *Dependent List* and—if desired—any independent variable(s) for splitting the data set in the field *Factor List*. In the additional menu *Statistics*, we can set the desired precision (95% by default). The output then provides a whole series of descriptive statistics, including the confidence interval around the mean(s) (Fig. 6.6).

Descriptives

Area				Statistic	Std. Error
Yield	1	Mean		35.20	1.659
		95% Confidence Interval for Mean	Lower Bound	31.45	
			Upper Bound	38.95	

Fig. 6.6 Exemplary output of an exploratory data analysis with SPSS. This includes the mean and the bounds of the corresponding confidence intervals for all selected dependent variables, grouped according to the levels of the independent variables

Decision Errors, Effect Sizes, and Power

In Chap. 5, we have introduced several variants of the t-test. The general procedure of computing such tests is identical for all significance tests, however, and we therefore recapitulate it here.

We had started from the assumption that the H_0 was true—usually this hypothesis postulates the non-existence of a difference. If the empirical (or even more extreme) data are very unlikely under this assumption, however, we question the validity of the H_0: Instead, we decide to believe in the H_1 and speak of a significant result. To enable such decisions, we had first defined what "very unlikely" means, and this probability is the significance level α. From the data of a sample, we had then calculated an empirical t-value that comes with a known theoretical distribution—under the assumption that the H_0 is true, plus a few auxiliary assumptions. Now, in order to decide between the two hypotheses, we have introduced two possibilities. First, we can determine whether the empirical t-value is larger than a critical t-value, which depends, among other things, on the significance level α. Second, we can calculate an exact value for this probability: The p-value that most statistical programs readily provide in their output. A decision in favor of H_1 is made if the p-value is less than or equal to α. The p-value is thus the conditional probability of the data (or even more extreme data) assuming that the H_0 is true, that is, $p = P(\text{data}|H_0)$.

Although significant results are often desired (see also Box 7.1), we will see in the course of this chapter that mere significance does not yield direct information about the size of an effect. A relevant question is thus whether we should distinguish statistical significance from "substantive relevance" or "practical significance"? Moreover, we never know which hypothesis really is true in the population: All our decisions are subject to some uncertainty, and may actually be wrong. In this chapter, we will introduce the concepts needed to answer the above question and we start with classifying different statistical decisions and their associated decision errors.

© Springer-Verlag GmbH Germany, part of Springer Nature 2023
M. Janczyk, R. Pfister, *Understanding Inferential Statistics*,
https://doi.org/10.1007/978-3-662-66786-6_7

7.1   Decision Errors in Inferential Statistics

Statistical significance is merely a statement about probabilities: If there was no difference (effect) in the population, then our empirical or more extreme data are very unlikely (in other words, the probability of observing such outcome is less than or equal to α if the H_0 were true). Specifying an α level puts an upper bound to the uncertainty attached to any decision in favor of the H_1, but we cannot fully shield ourselves from making an incorrect decision (see also Sect. 4.2.3). Also: What do we do if the result of a test is not significant? With the methods introduced so far, we would not decide against the H_0 in this case— but explicitly deciding in favor of the H_0 does not seem to be warranted either, especially because we do not know anything about the certainty of such a decision yet. After all, the H_1 might still be true in the population, that is, there might actually be an effect. In this case we would erroneously stick with the H_0.

   We thus look at the following situation: In the population either H_0 or H_1 is true, and we ultimately decide in favor of one of the two hypotheses on the basis of the significance test. This results in a pattern of correct and incorrect decisions as is shown in Fig. 7.1 (see also Sect. 4).

   Type I errors refer to a (wrong) decision in favor of the H_1 although the H_0 is true in the population. We would thus believe in an effect that does not actually exist. The procedures discussed so far explicitly control this error by allowing it to occur with a probability of α (therefore this error is sometimes called α-error). **Type II errors** refer to a (wrong) decision to stick with the H_0, although the H_1 is true in the population. This error type thus implies a failure to detect an existing effect. So far, we cannot say anything about the probability of this error; in analogy to the α-error, this wrong decision is also called β-error and the associated probability is referred to as β.

Decision for...	Actually true is...	
	H_0	H_1
H_0	correct	Type II error
H_1	Type I error	correct

Fig. 7.1 Correct and incorrect decisions in hypothesis testing

In Depth 7.1: Significance, Replication, Publication Bias

As we have seen, a true effect in the population does not necessarily translate into a "significant result" when conducting an empirical study. Conversely, "significant results" can also occur when there is *no* effect in the population. This state of affairs implies that any of the effects reported in the scientific literature do not necessarily have to be replicated in a follow-up study—whether replications succeed does not only depend on whether or not an effect exists, but also on such factors as the corresponding effect size and the sample size used in the new study. Last, but certainly not least, it also depends on chance, because empirical data will always include random variation. This reasoning has also recently been used to critically evaluate published studies that suggest the existence of a particular effect: If many significant tests are reported in a study, even though each experiment has a comparatively high probability β for a Type II error, then one may reasonably doubt the validity of the results. One reason for such a pattern of results may be that "significant" results were selectively reported while omitting non-significant results, because reporting non-significant results often renders publication of a study more difficult ("publication bias"). In this context, systematic re-investigation with so-called "tests for excess significance" (Francis et al. 2014) is an example of how statistical analyses can help to assess the validity of research results (see also Simonsohn 2013). The pursuit and active search for significant results, which are then published, can quickly lead to a false picture of whether an effect actually exists or not (see also Simmons et al. 2011).

7.2 Effect Sizes

Let us briefly recapitulate the pair of two-sided hypotheses of the *t*-test (for independent samples):

$$H_0 : \mu_A = \mu_B \quad \text{and} \quad H_1 : \mu_A \neq \mu_B.$$

While the H_0 is formulated *exactly* (it holds only if both values are exactly identical; see Sect. 4.1.2), the H_1 is formulated *inexactly*. For example, with $\mu_B = 100$, the H_1 would be true for both $\mu_A = 1000$ and $\mu_A = 100.1$. In most cases we will have little reason to formulate an exact H_1, because we do not know the population parameters involved. However, for an important consideration in this context, see the following quote from Cohen (1990, p. 1308):

A little thought reveals a fact widely understood among statisticians: The null hypothesis, taken literally (and that's the only way you can take it in formal hypothesis testing), is *always*

false in the real world. It can only be true in the bowels of a computer processor running a
Monte Carlo study (and even then a stray electron can make it false). If it is false, even to a
tiny degree, it must be the case that a large enough sample will produce a significant result
and lead to its rejection. So if the null hypothesis is always false, what's the big deal about
rejecting it?" (emphasis in original).

In other words, this statement says that, if we just make the samples large enough, we
will likely get a significant test result even if $\mu_B = 100$ and $\mu_A = 100.001$ (or at even
smaller differences). However, this small difference between μ_A and μ_B may be of so little
practical use or meaning that the statistical significance of the difference does not matter
any longer.

Let us now consider the (unknown) difference in the expected values of the populations,
that is, $\mu_A - \mu_B$. This difference comes with a troubling property: Its numerical magnitude
depends on the unit in which the variables are measured. Therefore, we standardize this
difference relative to the standard deviation of the populations and denote the resulting
difference as δ (a small delta) (see Cohen 1988). This quantity δ is an example of a so-
called **effect size**:

$$\delta = \frac{\mu_A - \mu_B}{\sigma}. \tag{7.1}$$

Of course, we do not know the value of δ, since it is again a population parameter.
However, if two samples already exist from the populations of interest A and B, we can
estimate the effect with

$$d = \frac{M_A - M_B}{\hat{\sigma}}. \tag{7.2}$$

Depending on whether the two samples are independent or dependent, $\hat{\sigma}$ has to be
calculated differently:

* *Independent samples:* In case of homogeneity of variance, the corrected variances
  of both samples are estimators for the same population variance. Therefore, both are
  pooled to obtain a better estimate for the population variance:

$$\hat{\sigma} = \sqrt{\frac{(n_A - 1)\hat{S}_A^2 + (n_B - 1)\hat{S}_B^2}{n_A + n_B - 2}}. \tag{7.3}$$

* *Dependent samples:* As with confidence intervals, the standard deviation of the
  difference values is used in this case (or the standard deviation of the raw values in
  the one-sample case):

$$\hat{\sigma} = \hat{S}_D. \tag{7.4}$$

With δ we now have a method to compare the observed effects of multiple studies—at least if their designs allow for calculating a t-test. Of course, there are also corresponding measures of effect sizes for other experimental designs, and we will get acquainted with some more of them in the following chapters (for a detailed account, see, e.g., Rosnow and Rosenthal 2003). To judge whether an observed effect is strong enough to be substantively relevant, it is helpful to know what a "small" effect or a "large" effect is. Statistics cannot provide an answer to this—but there are (more or less) accepted conventions. According to the most influential proposal $d = 0.2$ is a small, $d = 0.5$ a medium, and $d = 0.8$ a large effect (Cohen 1988).[1]

In Depth 7.2: Cohen's d and its Variants

The effect size presented here is often labeled as Cohen's d_s (for independent samples) or Cohen's d_z (for dependent samples) in the research literature and it is directly related to the corresponding t-test (Cohen 1988). In addition, numerous other formulas exist for calculating effect sizes for this situation. These other measures differ primarily in the standard deviation used in Formulas 7.3 and 7.4 and suggest using standard deviations that do not correspond to the variance used for the t-test. For example, the estimate of variance used in Formula 7.3 assumes homogeneity of variance. If this cannot be assumed, there are alternatives known as Hedges g or Glass's Δ, whereas alternative methods for Formula 7.4 take into account the correlation of the measurements (for an overview, see Ellis 2010, or Goulet-Pelletier and Cousineau 2018). Some authors recommend reporting these alternatives, since the measure d_z can be calculated from the t-statistic and the associated sample size, and is in a sense redundant (e.g., Lakens 2013). However, a main function of effect sizes is to enable power analyses for planning future studies (see Sect. 7.3), and power analyses for t-tests for dependent samples typically use the measure d_z. We therefore consider reporting precisely this measure to be useful and convenient for researchers that build on published findings. In each case, however, it should be specified which measure of effect size is being reported in order to allow correct interpretation.

---

[1] The procedure described in Formula 7.4 corresponds to the proposal of Cohen (1988). Furthermore, Cohen recommends using a corrected effect $d_c = d\sqrt{2}$ when calculating power (see Sect. 7.3) for dependent samples, and many computer programs automatically take this correction into account. Some authors go further to suggest reporting d_c as effect size instead of d, while other authors describe an adaptation of the conventions for interpreting effect sizes in case of dependent samples (Bortz 2005; Dunlap et al. 1996; Eid et al. 2010).

7.3   Power and the Type II Error

Effect sizes thus tell us something about the (standardized) size of an effect and they thus make different studies comparable by providing this standardized metric. Furthermore, they play an important role for determining β, the probability of committing a Type II error.

So far, we had only formulated the H_0 exactly, and this is necessary for determining the distribution (i.e., the probability density function) of the corresponding random variable (up to now this has always been t). This in turn was necessary to calculate the p-value as a conditional probability $p = P(\text{data}|H_0)$.

What about $P(\text{data}|H_1)$? According to the previous considerations, this probability cannot be determined, because the H_1 was always formulated inexactly. Determining a probability density function for a test statistic, however, requires an exactly formulated hypothesis: After all, there is an infinite number of possible alternative hypotheses, and the probability density function would look different for each of these possibilities. To avoid this, however, the H_1 can be formulated exactly, for example, by postulating "μ_A should be three measurement units larger than μ_B". In that case, we can derive the probability density function and, subsequently, we can determine the probability of interest.

Remember the t-test for independent samples: The H_0 states $\mu_A = \mu_B$ and we have said above that, assuming that the H_0 is true, the random variable that assigns to each pair of two samples a certain value t (see Formula 5.1), follows a t-distribution with $n_A + n_B - 2$ degrees of freedom as the probability density function. Here, the null hypothesis is used to determine the probability density function, and strictly speaking we are looking at a *central t-distribution*. Now what if the H_1 is true instead? Figure 7.2 illustrates the situation of two normally distributed variables under an exact alternative hypothesis, namely $H_1 : \mu_A = 0$

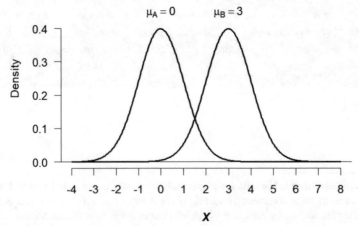

Fig. 7.2 Probability density functions in case of an alternative hypothesis $H_1 : \delta = 3$ (with $\sigma^2 = 1$)

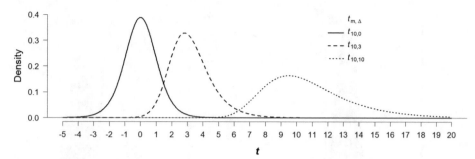

Fig. 7.3 Central t-distribution (i.e., with non-centrality parameter $\Delta = 0$; solid line), and two examples for non-central t-distributions with $\Delta = 3$ (dashed line) and $\Delta = 10$ (dotted line). All three probability density functions have $m = 10$ degrees of freedom

and $\mu_B = 3$ or $H_1 : \mu_B = \mu_A + 3$. For simplicity, let us assume $\sigma^2 = 1$. We can then write the hypotheses as follows:

$$H_0 : \delta = 0 \qquad \text{and} \qquad H_1 : \delta = 3.$$

In this situation (just as with any other H_1), the t-ratio no longer follows a central t-distribution, however, but rather is **non-centrally t-distributed.** To describe the corresponding probability density function, we need the so-called **non-centrality parameter** Δ (an uppercase Delta) as an additional parameter. In simple terms, Δ depends on the effect size δ that underlies the corresponding H_1: With increasing δ, Δ becomes larger as well. Figure 7.3 illustrates the effect of this parameter relative to a central t-distribution with ten degrees of freedom (the solid line). The figure includes two non-central t-distributions with ten degrees of freedom (for $\Delta = 3$ and $\Delta = 10$). We can see (1) that the non-central probability density function is no longer symmetric around zero, (2) that it becomes wider, and (3) that it is steeper on the left-hand side than on the right-hand side.

How can we now use non-central distributions to learn something about β, the probability of committing a Type II error? In the left panel of Fig. 7.4, we have our familiar situation again: The test statistic t is centrally t-distributed when assuming the H_0 (with ten degrees of freedom in the example). In addition, we have plotted the critical t-value for $\alpha = 0.05$ (for the case of a one-sided test). Thus, the red area is exactly 5% of the total area under the probability density function and the green area is 95% of the total area (see also Fig. 4.2). If an empirical t-value is larger than t_{crit}, we would reject the H_0 and believe in the H_1 instead (i.e., we would have obtained a significant result).

The right panel of Fig. 7.4 additionally shows the non-central t-distribution with a non-centrality parameter $\Delta = 3$. This is the probability density function of the t-value when both samples were drawn from populations with different μs, that is, when a certain H_1 is true in the population. The blue area (denoted $1 - \beta$), that is, the area to the right of t_{crit} under the non-central probability density function, is the probability of obtaining

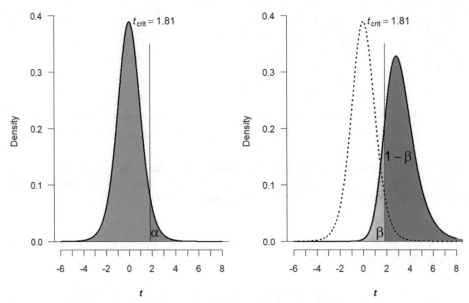

Fig. 7.4 The left panel shows a central t-distribution under the assumption that the H_0 is true, and the right panel displays an additional non-central t-distribution under the assumption that the H_1 is true (with non-centrality parameter $\Delta = 3$). In both figures, the probability density functions have $m = 10$ degrees of freedom

an empirical t-value larger than t_{crit} *if* this particular H_1 is true in the population. In other words, the blue area is the probability of getting a significant result if indeed this particular H_1 is true. And it is precisely this probability that we call **power**, which is also written as $1 - \beta$. In Cohen's words (1988, p. 4):

> *"The power of a statistical test of a null hypothesis is the probability that it will lead to the rejection of the null hypothesis,* i. e., *the probability that it will result in the conclusion that the phenomenon exists."* (emphasis in original).

The orange area β, that is, the area under the non-central distribution from $-\infty$ to t_{crit}, is the probability of getting an empirical t-value that leads us to continue believing in the null hypothesis (i.e., to a non-significant result) *despite* the H_1 being true. This case is exactly what we referred to above as a Type II error. Thus, if we know the power of a test, we can also determine the probability of committing a Type II error.

In reality though, we usually do not know the power of a test, because we usually cannot know how large the effect is in the population—but this would be required for an exact formulation of the H_1 (and, as a consequence, is what determines the non-centrality parameter). We now consider what factors influence the power:

- *Choice of significance level α:* The critical t-value is, of course, related to α. It becomes smaller the larger α is. In other words: If we choose a larger α (i.e., we accept a larger probability of a Type I error), we make it "easier" to obtain a significant result. From the left panel of Fig. 7.4 it becomes clear that by choosing a larger value for α, the red area becomes larger. At the same time, the blue area (the power) in the right panel of Fig. 7.4 also becomes larger while the orange area (β) becomes smaller. Thus, the probabilities for Type I and Type II errors behave in opposite ways.

- *"True" effect size:* The larger the effect in the population is, the larger the non-centrality parameter becomes. As a consequence, the non-central t-distribution moves to the right (see Fig. 7.3). Since the critical t-value does not change, the power becomes larger just as well.

- Furthermore, reducing the relevant standard error increases power. Because the standard error is in the denominator of the t-ratio, the t-value becomes larger with a smaller standard error and the power of the test thus increases. Such a reduction can, on the one hand, result from a *smaller population variance*, since the variances of the samples then tend to become smaller as well (and these are in the numerator of the standard error). On the other hand, smaller standard errors can result from *increasing the sample size*, which is in the denominator of the standard error.

How can this information be useful to us? Most of the time, we do not know the "true" size of the effect and therefore cannot specify it. However, there are two possible ways to specify an effect, and thus the H_1: (1) We can estimate the population effect from the results of previous studies on a similar topic, or (2) we can define a minimum effect size of interest. For practical considerations, we might, for example, only be interested in statistically detecting a "large" effect, while smaller effects are practically not relevant and therefore need not be detected at all. We also have only little if any influence on the population variance, but it is possible to reduce the relevant standard error by increasing the sample size. As this increases the power, it also increases the chances of obtaining a significant result.

7.4 Optimal Sample Size

We have discussed four variables in this chapter as summarized in Fig. 7.5. These four variables are interdependent: If we know three of them, we can determine the fourth. These components form the framework of Neyman and Pearson's concept of hypothesis testing (see Box 4.2). Furthermore, we can now express the key point from the above quote of Cohen as follows:

> The larger the sample size, the higher the power of a test.

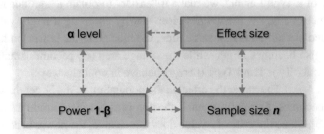

Fig. 7.5 The four interdependent variables in the framework of statistical hypothesis testing

Thus, if the sample size n approaches infinity ($n \rightarrow \infty$), we are almost guaranteed to obtain a significant result, that is, the power also approaches 1. We should therefore ask the following critical question: Is it always desirable to aim for maximally large samples? This question usually receives a negative answer, and there are at least three good reasons for this:

- Organizational and institutional reasons often speak against this: We cannot recruit infinitely many participants and/or spend an infinite amount of (financial) resources on a single study.
- If the power approaches 1, even tiny effects would become statistically significant, even though they might be practically irrelevant and can therefore safely be "overlooked".
- Moreover, the power does not increase linearly with the sample size. Rather, it initially increases steeply with increasing n, but this increase becomes progressively flatter and then approaches 1 in an asymptotic fashion (see Fig. 7.6). In other words, increasing the sample size from $n = 10$ to $n = 50$ has a large impact on the power of a study; however, further increasing the sample size to $n = 100$ will only yield a modest increase in power. The comparison of independent and dependent samples in Fig. 7.6 further illustrates a decisive advantage of dependent samples with respect to power, which we will return to in Sect. 10.3.

Against this background, it does not seem very useful to aim for maximally large samples. A reasoning along the following lines is preferable instead:

Based on (practical) considerations, we could determine for a planned study that we are only interested in effects of a particular size, for example, only in "large" effects of $\delta = 0.8$. Because we do not want to presuppose a particular direction of the effect, we plan to use a two-sided t-test for two independent samples as the significance test. Furthermore, we choose a probability of $\alpha = 0.05$ for Type I errors. If an effect of at least the assumed size is actually present in the population, we want to detect it with a probability of 80%, that is, $1 - \beta = 0.8$.

Thus, three of the four variables in Fig. 7.5 are determined, and the fourth—the optimal sample size n—can then be calculated. There is no easy way to perform this calculation

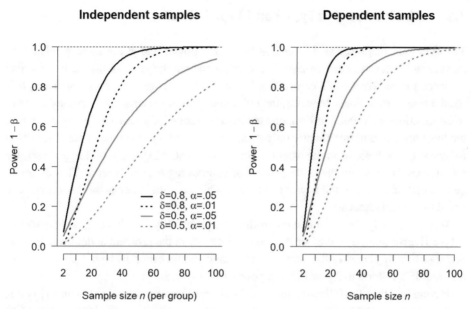

Fig. 7.6 Illustration of the power as a function of sample size for the case of a *t*-test with independent samples (left panel) and dependent samples (right panel). Compared to the solid lines, for the dashed lines the value of α is reduced; for the red lines, a smaller effect δ was assumed

manually, but luckily there are three simple ways to determine the optimal value of n with corresponding tools:

- In the classical variant, we could use the book by Cohen (1988). This book contains a large number of tables for determining the power or optimal sample size for various types of tests.
- A more modern variant is offered by the freely available program G*Power (Faul et al. 2007). G*Power offers flexible options for power analyses, determining optimal sample size, and graphical illustration of the resulting situations.
- Furthermore, power analyses can also be performed with R as we will describe in Sect. 7.6.1. For more details in case of within-subject designs (including more complicated cases than considered so far), see also Langenberg et al. (2022).

In the above situation, all variants suggest an optimal sample size of $n = 26$ per group. If we had been looking for a "medium effect", each group would be of size $n = 64$, and for a "small effect", the optimal sample size is already $n = 394$ per group.

7.5   The Interplay of Type I and Type II Error

The definition of power as $1 - \beta$ highlights that power and β are closely related. In most cases, researchers are interested in rejecting the null hypothesis, that is, in obtaining evidence for an effect while controlling for the probability of a Type I error. Thus, α is fixed a priori. Sometimes, however, the null hypothesis is the research hypothesis, and in these situations we require information about the certainty of a decision for the H_0. Using the tools presented in this chapter (effect size, power, and optimal sample size), we could follow a similar logic as in the example above: When sticking to the null hypothesis, we might want to constrain the probability β of committing a Type II error. This β can be determined, if we know the power of the test, which in turn depends on the sample size and the assumed effect size.

Whether a study should aim at controlling the probability of either a Type I error or of a Type II error (e.g., $\alpha = 0.05$ or $\beta = 0.05$), depends on the problem under investigation. A suggestion by Cohen (1988) states that the ratio should generally be $\alpha : \beta = 1 : 4$; for a $\alpha = 0.05$ it follows that $\beta = 0.2$ or a power $1 - \beta = 0.8$.

Having said this, the following relation should now be clear: Merely knowing a p-value that is reported in the context of empirical research does not tell much about the size of an effect. A result is either significant ($p \leq \alpha$) or not significant ($p > \alpha$). In order to judge a research result, it is always necessary to consider other characteristics: The type of test used, the empirical test value, the degrees of freedom of the test, and a measure of effect size are necessary to properly and comprehensively judge a result. In addition, manuscript guidelines also require the reporting of an effect size (APA 2020).

In Depth 7.3: Interpreting $p > .05$

Common significance tests focus on the null hypothesis and we calculate the p-value under the assumption that the H_0 is true. Significance tests thus focus primarily on the rejection of this hypothesis, because we know the probability of a Type I error in this situation: It corresponds to the α-level of the test, usually $\alpha = 0.05$. The probability for a decision not to reject the null hypothesis—β—on the other hand, cannot be readily determined in most cases (this would require an exactly formulated alternative hypothesis; see Sect. 7.3).

A decision rationale of "$p > \alpha$, so H_0 is true" therefore has to be treated with caution and should be discussed in conjunction with other characteristics such as the sample size used (because large samples allow high power and thus a low probability β). Especially in case of "almost significant results" such as $p = 0.051$,

---

(continued)

it is therefore advisable not to draw strong conclusions from this result. Instead, researchers are well advised to obtain further empirical evidence via additional studies in this case.

This procedure is particularly relevant when a study is planned with the aim of showing evidence for the equality of certain conditions or people, that is, to stick with the null hypothesis. Since in this case, no exact alternative hypothesis can be formulated, using a large α-level of, for example, $\alpha = 0.20$ is often recommended. Alternative approaches for this situation are so-called equivalence tests (Lakens 2017) or, in particular, Bayesian methods, which we present in Chap. 12.

7.6 Examples and Exercises

Effect sizes, such as d introduced in this chapter, are not contained in the default output of corresponding t-tests. In many cases, we will therefore have to calculate this statistic manually. We will illustrate this procedure in the following by using the formulas of this chapter. A helpful homepage with information and flexible online calculators is http://www.psychometrica.de/effect_size.html.

7.6.1 Effect Sizes with R

We again turn to the exemplary data on the yield of different barley fields at the Guinness Brewery (see also Sect. 5.5.1, Table 5.1 for independent samples and Table 5.2 for dependent samples).

- **Example 1:** First, we want to calculate the effect size for the comparison of the two areas from Table 5.1. We again assume that the data come in the form of two vectors: `yield` indicates the yield in arbitrary units, `area` indicates from which area the measured value originates. According to Formula 7.2, we first calculate the mean difference:

```
mdiff <- mean(yield[area == 1]) -
         mean(yield[area == 2])
```

In addition, we determine the standard deviation of the difference. To do this, we first compute the sample sizes and the (corrected) standard deviations:[2]

```
n_a <- length(yield[area == 1])
n_b <- length(yield[area == 2])
s_a <- sd(yield[area == 1])
s_b <- sd(yield[area == 2])
```

We can then determine the standard deviation of the difference from the calculated variables (see Formula 7.3), and together with the mean difference, we can calculate d:

```
sddiff <- sqrt(((n_a-1)*s_a^2 + (n_b-1)*s_b^2)
                / (n_a+n_b-2))
d <- mdiff / sddiff
d

1.469161
```

Accordingly, there is a very large effect. Together with the result of the t-tests from Sect. 5.5.1, we can now fully report the observed difference between the two areas, $t(18) = 3.29, p = .004, d = 1.47$.

- **Example 2:** To calculate the effect size for a comparison of two dependent samples, we use the data from Table 5.2. Here, fields were treated with different fertilizers in two consecutive years. The mean difference can be calculated as:

```
mdiff <- mean(yield_2013) - mean(yield_2012)
```

We then determine the pairwise differences and their standard deviation:

```
fertilizer_effect <- yield_2013 - yield_2012
sddiff <- sd(fertilizer_effect)
```

The effect size can then be calculated using Formulas 7.2 and 7.4:

```
d <- mdiff / sddiff
d

0.743614
```

The fertilizer thus not only has a significant influence on the yield of the fields, but the influence is also reflected as an effect of medium size, $t(9) = 2.35, p = .022$, $d = 0.74$.

---

[2] An elegant alternative to this procedure is to take the standard deviation of the difference directly from the output of t.test(). The corresponding syntax is described in the online material. Direct access to effect sizes is also provided by various R packages such as compute.es or MBESS.

Note that the function `t_out()` when applied to the *t*-test for dependent samples does not, by default, report the corrected effect size $d_c = d\sqrt{2}$ (see also Footnote 2 in this chapter; in this case $d_c = 1.05$). In order to obtain the corrected effect size, we would have to use the argument `d.corr = TRUE`:

```
library(schoRsch)
t_out( t.test(...), d.corr = TRUE)
```

- **Example 3:** In Example 1, we had calculated an effect size of $d = 1.47$. We can now use this to estimate the power achieved in this study. To do this, we use the function `power.t.test()`, to which we pass the size of both samples and the effect size:

```
power.t.test(n = 10, delta = 1.47, sd = 1,
             type = "two.sample",
             alternative = "two.sided")

Two-sample t test power calculation

             n = 10
         delta = 1.47
            sd = 1
     sig.level = 0.05
         power = 0.8743837
   alternative = two.sided
```

The output returns a power estimate of 0.87. Thus, if we assume the observed effect size as the true effect size, there is—to put it simply—a probability of 87% to detect an effect of this size as significant with samples of the size $n = 10$ (at a significance level $\alpha = 0.05$ and for a non-directional alternative hypothesis; for the interpretation of $1 - \beta = 0.87$, see also Box 5.4).

7.6.2 Effect Sizes with SPSS

For the calculation with SPSS, we also turn back to the data on the yield of different barley fields of the Guinness Brewery (see Sect. 5.5.2, Table 5.3 for independent samples and Table 5.4 for dependent samples).

- **Example 1:** First, we would like to calculate the effect size for the comparison of the two areas from Table 5.3. For these data, we now calculate a *t*-test for independent samples and can take all necessary values from its results table in the output (see Fig. 5.3). These values are then fed into the corresponding formulas (mean values, corrected standard deviations, sample size). According to Formula 7.3 we calculate

$$\hat{\sigma} = \sqrt{\frac{(10-1)\cdot 5.245^2 + (10-1)\cdot 6.027^2}{10+10-2}} = 5.650,$$

and with Formula 7.2, the effect size d is calculated as:

$$d = \frac{35.2 - 26.9}{5.650} = 1.469,$$

Together with the results of the t-tests from Sect. 5.5.2, we can now fully report the observed difference between the two areas, $t(18) = 3.29$, $p = .004$, $d = 1.47$.

- **Example 2:** Now we want to calculate the effect size in case of dependent samples, using the data from Table 5.4. First, we calculate the mean values of the two variables `yield_2012` and `yield_2013` via the menu

`Analyze > Descriptive Statistics > Descriptives...`

Then, we calculate the difference values of the two variables and analyze this new variable with a t-test for one sample. This procedure can be seen in Example 3 of the exercises for SPSS in Chap. 5. Now we can take all values from the two result tables and enter them into Formulas 7.2 and 7.4. According to Formula 7.4 we obtain

$$\hat{\sigma} = 3.093,$$

and with Formula 7.2, the effect size is calculated as

$$d = \frac{29.2 - 26.9}{3.093} = 0.744.$$

Together with the results of the t-test from Sect. 5.5.2, we can now describe the difference completely, $t(9) = 2.35$, $p = 0.022$, $d = 0.74$. Accordingly, there is a significant effect of medium size.

One-Way Analysis of Variance (ANOVA)

The methods introduced in the preceding chapters enable us to evaluate difference hypotheses for up to two groups or conditions with t-tests. Many actual research designs will include more than two groups or conditions, however, and these situations require a different statistical approach.

To illustrate such cases, we will use a new example here and in the following chapters: A researcher is interested in whether memory performance is affected by one or two days of sleep deprivation. To allow for a clear-cut interpretation, this researcher also wants to assess normal, baseline performance. This design translates to three conditions: One control group without any sleep deprivation, one group with one day (and night) of sleep deprivation and another group with two days (and nights) of sleep deprivation. The three conditions will thus be implemented in three independent groups. Participants have to learn a list of 40 words and we analyze how many of these words can be recalled after a certain amount of time as the dependent variable.

We will use analysis of variance (ANOVA) to test whether there are differences in the means of the three populations underlying these groups. In this chapter, we introduce the easiest version of this procedure. This version applies to research designs with only one independent variable, but this independent variable can have more than two levels. In a sense, it thus generalizes the t-tests for two independent samples to more than two groups. Independent variables are usually called *factors* in ANOVA terminology, hence the name of **one-way or single-factor ANOVA**. Building on this, we consider more complex ANOVA versions in the two following chapters.

© Springer-Verlag GmbH Germany, part of Springer Nature 2023
M. Janczyk, R. Pfister, *Understanding Inferential Statistics*,
https://doi.org/10.1007/978-3-662-66786-6_8

8.1   ANOVA: Basic Concepts

8.1.1   Why ANOVA? α-Inflation and α-Adjustment

Why do we actually need a new test? Could we not simply compare all three combinations of two groups by computing three separate t-tests, that is, group 1 vs. 2, 1 vs. 3, and 2 vs. 3? Even though such a strategy seems intuitive, it comes with the problem of increasing the probability of erroneous decisions. This problem of **α-inflation** (or **α-cumulation**) is our main focus in this section.

The core of the problem is that—as discussed in the previous chapters—any hypothesis test can be significant "by chance" and thus lead to a Type I error. Suppose we were to run k tests on the same α-level, while the H_0 is actually true for all tests: What is the probability that at least one of these tests randomly (and thus erroneously) shows a significant result? We will see that this probability is not equal to the individual α-level, but it is systematically larger.

We can use the so-called binomial distribution to calculate the probability of observing at least one significant test when running a total series of k tests, if we assume the H_0 to be true and decide for any given α:

$$P(m \geq 1) = 1 - P(m = 0) = 1 - (1 - \alpha)^k. \tag{8.1}$$

Now recall the example from the beginning of this chapter. To compare all three conditions (no sleep deprivation vs. 1 day of sleep deprivation vs. 2 days of sleep deprivation), we would need $k = 3$ t-tests. Further, we use $\alpha = .05$ and assume that the null hypothesis is true in all cases. Plugging these values into Formula 8.1 yields:

$$P(m \geq 1) = 1 - (1 - .05)^3 = 0.14.$$

Hence, the probability of at least one erroneous decision with this procedure is already about three times as large as the chosen α level.

A way to circumvent this issue is called **α-adjustment**: Each individual test uses an adjusted α' so that the cumulative probability of at least one decision error does not exceed α. A useful and common approximation to determine α' is the **Bonferroni correction:**

$$\alpha' = \frac{\alpha}{k}.$$

For our example, the new α would be $\alpha' = 0.01\overline{6}$ and according to Formula 8.1, this yields a probability of 0.049 for at least one erroneous decision—even slightly less than the original $\alpha = 0.05$. The Bonferroni correction is thus a conservative correction. Using this correction lets us err on the side of caution, while accepting reduced power. ANOVA avoids the problem of α-inflation while retaining statistical power.

In Depth 8.1: α-Inflation in Physiological Studies
As outlined in the main text, erroneous decisions in favor of the H_1 are more likely, the more non-adjusted tests we calculate. This is particularly evident in the analysis of neurophysiological data. Functional magnetic resonance imaging (fMRI) studies, for example, often perform t-tests evaluating each voxel of the brain (also called mass-univariate testing). A voxel is a small unit of volume; a cube with edges of about 2 mm in length. Covering a whole brain worth of voxels thus easily leads to 10,000 or more independent tests. Computing this many tests without adequate α-adjustments can produce peculiar outcomes so that, for example, systematic activation patterns seemingly emerge even in the brain of a dead salmon (Bennett et al. 2011)—a clear example why multiple tests require appropriate corrections.

8.1.2 Terminology, Hypotheses, and Assumptions

In the context of ANOVA, an independent variable is usually called a **factor** and its values are called **levels (of the factor)**. The study in the introductory example, therefore, has one factor "sleep deprivation" with three levels. The number of words recalled is the dependent variable.

Factors are not limited to three levels, of course, and we will denote the (unspecified) number of factor levels with J. Each of these factor levels is associated with a population from which the corresponding sample is drawn. Similar to the t-test for two independent samples, we assume that the samples are drawn *independently of one another*. Since the samples are not necessarily of the same size, we denote their size by n_j. We can now use this terminology to describe the structure of our data as shown in Table 8.1: Each y_{ij} represents a single data point (e.g., the measured dependent variable for a participant), the index i denotes the number of the data point within a factor level, and the index j indicates the corresponding factor level.

Table 8.1 Design and terminology for the one-way ANOVA. The index i refers to the participant within a group and the index j refers to the group itself

Level 1	$\cdots$	Level j	$\cdots$	Level J
y_{11}	$\cdots$	y_{1j}	$\cdots$	y_{1J}
$\vdots$		$\vdots$		$\vdots$
y_{i1}	$\cdots$	y_{ij}	$\cdots$	y_{iJ}
$\vdots$		$\vdots$		$\vdots$
y_{n_11}	$\cdots$	y_{n_jj}	$\cdots$	y_{n_JJ}

Further, we denote our dependent variable by Y_j and assume that it is measured (at least) at interval scale level when sampling from the population j. As with the t-test, we assume that the dependent variable is normally distributed in each population with identical variance σ^2 (homogeneity of variance). Mathematically, these assumptions can be summarized as follows:

$$Y_j \sim N(\mu_j, \sigma^2) \qquad \forall j \in \{1, \ldots, J\}. \tag{8.2}$$

Since the one-way ANOVA discussed here generalizes the t-test for two independent samples, the corresponding H_0 is also a generalization of the H_0 as discussed for the t-test. The H_1 essentially states that the H_0 is not true. Accordingly, the two hypotheses are formulated as:

$$H_0 : \quad \mu_1 = \mu_2 = \ldots = \mu_J \quad \text{and}$$

$$H_1 : \quad \mu_k \neq \mu_m \text{ for at least one pair } k, m \in \{1, \ldots, J\}.$$

In other words, the H_1 states that at least two of the population means are not equal. Importantly, it does not state that *all* population means are different from one another, already one pairwise difference is sufficient for this hypothesis to be true.

8.1.3 The Rationale of ANOVA

In this section, we will elaborate on the idea behind ANOVA and on how to construct an appropriate test statistic in this context. We will again use the introductory example and assume that we have collected a sample for each of the three conditions. In Fig. 8.1, we have plotted three hypothetical sample means obtained in this way in two versions. The error bars represent hypothetical variances of the dependent variable in the population, which is larger in the left panel than in the right panel of Fig. 8.1. The following intuitive argument for the construction of a test statistic consists of two steps:

- The more different the sample means are, the more strongly do the data speak against the H_0, which assumes equality of all population means. To capture this difference formally, we can calculate the variance of the sample means: The larger this variance, the more different the means are, and the more the data speak against the H_0.
- The sample means (and hence their variability around an overall mean) are identical in both panels of Fig. 8.1. Arguably, however, given differences between means speak more against the H_0 when the variance of the dependent variable in the population is small, that is, in the right panel of Fig. 8.1.

    We will use simulations to demonstrate that this intuition is indeed correct. That is, the simulations will show that differences between means increase as the variance within the underlying population increases. Let us start with the simple case of two

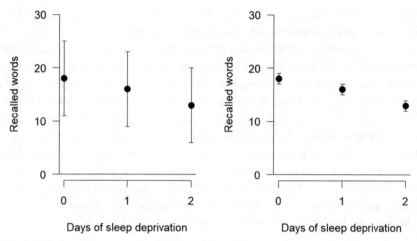

Fig. 8.1 Identical sample means for three conditions. The error bars represent the variance of the dependent variable in the population, which is larger in the left panel than in the right panel

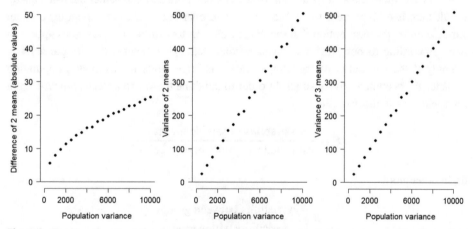

Fig. 8.2 Results of a simulation to illustrate the effect of the population variance of the dependent variable on the difference between two means (left panel) and its influence on the variance of two means (middle panel) or three means (right panel)

means, because we can simply calculate the difference in this case. We have assumed populations with different variances (from 500 to 10,000 in steps of 500 arbitrary units). For each of these population variances, we then sampled 1000 sets of two samples ($n =$ 20), calculated the absolute value of the mean difference, and averaged the difference across the 1000 samples. The result is shown in the left panel of Fig. 8.2. Indeed, the difference in means increases with the population variance. In other words, the larger the variance in the underlying population, the larger will be the difference between the means of samples from that population (on average). This happens even if all samples are drawn from the same population, that is, if the H_0 was true as in the simulations.

With more than two samples, a simple difference cannot be calculated to quantify the difference between means. We can calculate the variance of the means instead, however. With only two samples, their variance is the smaller the smaller the mean difference is. This is illustrated in the middle panel of Fig. 8.2, where we have calculated the variance of the two means and see that it also increases with the underlying population variance. Finally, the right panel of Fig. 8.2 brings us closer to the situation depicted in Fig. 8.1. Here, we have drawn three (instead of two) samples. Again, we see that the variance also increases with the underlying population variance. In sum, because large variances of the means are more likely to occur if the population variance is large, we also need to consider the variance of the dependent variable in the population. According to the above-mentioned assumptions (Formula 8.2), each of the (corrected) sample variances actually is an estimator for the same population variance σ^2. Hence, we will use the individual sample variances to construct a joint estimator $\hat{\sigma}^2$ for σ^2.

In Sect. 5.1, we have introduced two properties of test statistics with the example of the t-ratio: (1) The more the data speak against the H_0, the more extreme values the test statistic should take, and (2) we need to be able to derive the distribution of a corresponding random variable under the assumption that the H_0 is true. We now follow an analogous approach here: According to our previous considerations, data speak against the H_0 particularly strongly if the variability of the sample means is large while the estimated population variance σ^2 is comparatively small. In order to combine these two aspects, we will use a ratio that we call the **F-ratio**:

$$F = \frac{\text{variability of sample means}}{\text{estimated variability in population}},$$

or, in other words:

$$F = \frac{\text{variability between groups}}{\text{variability within groups}}.$$

A slightly different view emerges when considering the sources of these two variabilities:[1]

- The variability between groups is due to differences between the means of the groups. These differences reflect (1) (possible) differences between the corresponding population parameters (i.e., *effects of the factor*) and (2) *measurement error* (including population variability; see Fig. 8.2).

---

[1] We will see in Sect. 8.2.1 that the formulas for quantifying variability are very similar to the formula for variance. However, because it is not exactly the variance that is calculated, we prefer to use variability as general term here.

- Within each group, measurements are subject to some variability even in the absence of any effect. This variability is solely the result of *measurement errors* and population variability.

We can therefore also interpret the F-ratio as

$$F = \frac{\text{variability between groups}}{\text{variability within groups}} = \frac{\text{effects + measurement error}}{\text{measurement error}}.$$

This formulation highlights a typical (and desirable) behavior of the F-ratio: In the absence of effects (i.e., effects $= 0$), we will get $F = 1$, whereas we will get $F > 1$ if there are systematic effects. The F-ratio, therefore, becomes larger the stronger the effects are, that is, the more the data speak against the H_0. *Note:* Because different estimates of measurement error are used in the numerator and denominator, the F-ratio can also take values between 0 and 1 in practice.

In summary, the F-ratio satisfies at least one of the desired properties of a test statistic. If we also knew its distribution (i.e., the probability density function of an appropriate random variable), it would indeed be suitable as a test statistic in ANOVA. We will return to this distribution in Sect. 8.2.3.

8.2   Calculating ANOVA Statistics: A Hands-On Example

In this section, we will specify the computational steps involved in computing an ANOVA using the terminology introduced in Sect. 8.1.2. We illustrate the procedure with fictitious data for the introductory example as shown in Table 8.2. Here, each of the three groups comprises ten participants, that is, $n_1 = n_2 = n_3 = 10$. According to the means of the three groups, performance deteriorates with increasing sleep deprivation. (The numbers in parentheses after each value denote the age of the participants in years. We will ignore this information for now, but we will return to the example in Chap. 9 and take this additional variable into account).

Group means and variances can be calculated as usual according to Formulas 1.2 and 1.3—we only need to be mindful to perform separate calculations per group which we will denote by corresponding indices. Hence, within each group, the corresponding *group mean M_j* is calculated as

$$M_j = \frac{1}{n_j} \sum_{i=1}^{n_j} y_{ij} \qquad \forall j \in \{1, \ldots, J\}$$

Table 8.2 Exemplary data to illustrate the computational steps involved in ANOVA. The values correspond to the number of correctly recalled words in a memory test, and the number in parentheses indicates the age of the participants. We will focus on memory performance here, whereas the additional variable age becomes relevant in Chap. 9

Sleep deprivation		
0 days	1 day	2 days
22 (23 yrs.)	18 (19 yrs.)	17 (20 yrs.)
17 (51 yrs.)	15 (60 yrs.)	12 (56 yrs.)
19 (19 yrs.)	17 (24 yrs.)	16 (23 yrs.)
18 (27 yrs.)	16 (37 yrs.)	15 (21 yrs.)
14 (33 yrs.)	16 (18 yrs.)	13 (35 yrs.)
18 (43 yrs.)	15 (45 yrs.)	11 (45 yrs.)
16 (50 yrs.)	14 (57 yrs.)	10 (41 yrs.)
19 (61 yrs.)	16 (53 yrs.)	8 (51 yrs.)
20 (43 yrs.)	13 (44 yrs.)	13 (44 yrs.)
18 (21 yrs.)	17 (26 yrs.)	16 (36 yrs.)
M_j 18.1	15.7	13.1
S_j^2 4.29	2.01	7.69

and the group variance S_j^2 is calculated as

$$S_j^2 = \frac{1}{n_j} \sum_{i=1}^{n_j} (y_{ij} - M_j)^2 \qquad \forall j \in \{1, \ldots, J\}.$$

The resulting three means and variances are given in Table 8.2. Finally, we need to calculate the *grand mean* of all observations. With N as the total number of observations (i.e., $N = n_1 + n_2 + n_3 = 30$; resp. more generally: $N = \sum_{j=1}^{J} n_j$), the grand mean M is calculated as:

$$M = \frac{1}{N} \sum_{j=1}^{J} \sum_{i=1}^{n_j} y_{ij} \quad \text{or} \quad M = \sum_{j=1}^{J} \frac{n_j}{N} M_j. \tag{8.3}$$

According to the second formula, the grand mean M can also be understood as a *weighted average* of the group means M_j. Applied to the example, we get:

$$M = \sum_{j=1}^{3} \frac{n_j}{N} M_j = \frac{10}{30} \cdot 18.1 + \frac{10}{30} \cdot 15.7 + \frac{10}{30} \cdot 13.1 = 15.63.$$

8.2.1   Partitioning of Sums of Squares

After these initial computations, we now turn to an important mathematical concept in all ANOVAs: the so-called partitioning of the sums of squares. We will re-encounter this concept several times throughout the next chapters.

- First, we calculate the *total sum of squares*, which will be denoted as SS_{tot} in the following:

$$SS_{tot} = \sum_{j=1}^{J} \sum_{i=1}^{n_j} (y_{ij} - M)^2.$$

Here, the grand mean M is subtracted from each of the single observations, the result is squared, and everything is summed. Put differently, SS_{tot} is N-times the total variance. If one were to divide SS_{tot} by N, the result simply is the total variance of all data points. For our example, SS_{tot} is calculated as:

$$SS_{tot} = \sum_{j=1}^{3} \sum_{i=1}^{n_j} (y_{ij} - 15.63)^2$$

$$= (22 - 15.63)^2 + (17 - 15.63)^2 + \ldots + (13 - 15.63)^2 + (16 - 15.63)^2$$

$$= 264.97.$$

- As a second expression, we calculate the *sum of squares between the groups* (sometimes called *explained sum of squares*), which we denote as SS_A:[2]

$$SS_A = \sum_{j=1}^{J} n_j (M_j - M)^2. \tag{8.4}$$

Here, we subtract the grand mean from each group mean, square the result, multiply them with the respective sample size n_j, and sum up everything. Multiplying with sample size gives more weight to means from large samples than to those from small samples. We can thus conceptualize SS_A as a kind of weighted variance of the group means around the grand mean. Crucially, SS_A depends on actual effects and thus quantifies the influence of the factor (e.g., of an experimental manipulation). Applied

---

[2] It would perhaps be more intuitive to denote this sum of squares as SS_b (*b* for *between*). However, since we will also consider ANOVA with more than one factor in later chapters, we already introduce the index A at this point, and write SS_A to refer to the sum of squares that is due to the effects of the (here: only) factor A.

to the example, we get:

$$SS_A = \sum_{j=1}^{3} n_j (M_j - 15.63)^2$$

$$= 10 \cdot (18.1 - 15.63)^2 + 10 \cdot (15.7 - 15.63)^2 + 10 \cdot (13.1 - 15.63)^2$$

$$= 125.07.$$

- Finally, we can calculate the *sum of squares within the groups*, which we denote SS_w (*w* for *within*; this sum of squares is also often called *error/residual sum of squares* and denoted SS_{error}). In the one-way ANOVA considered here, it is also the basis for the error term that will be used in the denominator of the *F*-ratio:

$$SS_w = \sum_{j=1}^{J} \sum_{i=1}^{n_j} (y_{ij} - M_j)^2 = \sum_{j=1}^{J} n_j S_j^2. \tag{8.5}$$

According to the right part of the formula, the group variances are multiplied with their sample size and then added up. SS_w is also the basis for $\hat{\sigma}^2$, the estimator of the population variance. Applied to the example, we get:

$$SS_w = \sum_{j=1}^{3} n_j S_j^2 = 10 \cdot 4.29 + 10 \cdot 2.01 + 10 \cdot 7.69 = 139.90.$$

An important relationship between these three sums of squares is that SS_{tot} can be split—or: partitioned—into the other two sums of squares:

$$SS_{tot} = SS_A + SS_w.$$

This **partitioning of sums of squares** (or **partitioning of variance**) illustrates a basic principle of the ANOVA: The overall variability in the data is partitioned into parts that are due to differences between groups (here: SS_A), and parts that reflect the variability within groups (here: SS_w). The similarity of the sums of squares to variance also lends the ANOVA its name.

8.2.2   Mean Sums of Squares

The different sums of squares derive from different amounts of numerical values: While SS_w is calculated based on individual data points, SS_A is based on the means of the groups. This difference implies a different number of degrees of freedom. We can make the sums of squares comparable, however, by dividing them by their degrees of freedom. The resulting quantities are typically called **mean sums of squares**. Two such mean sums of squares are required to calculate the F-ratio:[3]

- SS_A has $J - 1$ degrees of freedom, therefore the *mean sum of squares between groups* is calculated as:

$$MS_A = \frac{SS_A}{J - 1}.$$

Thus, in our example, the result is:

$$MS_A = \frac{125.07}{3 - 1} = 62.53.$$

- SS_w has $N - J$ degrees of freedom (N again denotes the total number of observations), and the *mean sum of squares within groups* is calculated as:

$$MS_w = \frac{SS_w}{N - J}.$$

In the example, the result is:

$$MS_w = \frac{139.90}{30 - 3} = 5.18.$$

8.2.3   The *F*-Ratio and the *F*-Distribution

In a final step, we compute the (empirical) **F-ratio** or the (empirical) **F-value** as

$$F = \frac{MS_A}{MS_w},$$

and for our data from Table 8.2, the result is:

$$F = \frac{62.53}{5.18} = 12.07.$$

---

[3] In principle, there is also the mean sum of squares total (the corresponding degrees of freedom are $N - 1$). We will not need this value for the remaining calculations, however.

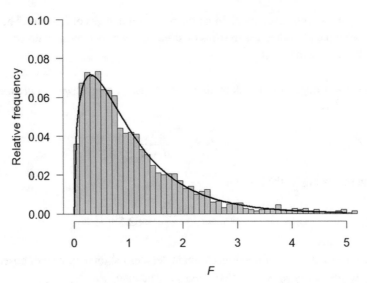

Fig. 8.3 Relative frequencies of F-values when drawing four samples of size $n = 10$ for 2000 times from the same normally distributed population

Now imagine that we draw J samples from a single population, that is, we assume the H_0 to be true, and we repeat this process infinitely many times. Then, from the data of each set of samples, we calculate the F-ratio and ask which values occur for F in this process. To illustrate, Fig. 8.3 shows the relative frequencies of such F-values for 2000 draws of four samples of size $n = 10$, each from the same normally distributed population (see Sect. 4.2 for a similar procedure in the case of two samples).

From Fig. 8.3 we see that negative F-values do not occur. This follows from how we have computed the numerator and denominator, which are both constructed from sums of squares. Furthermore, we see that the F-values are not distributed symmetrically around one particular value, as was the case with the normal distribution and the central t-distribution (see Fig. 4.2). However, assuming that the H_0 is true, the exact form of the distribution can be determined, which is the F-distribution: A random variable F that assigns to each combination of J samples the (empirical) F-value is F-distributed. Actually, assuming the H_0 to be true, it is the **central F-distribution**, which is again a whole family of distributions. Their exact shape is determined by two parameters, called the numerator and denominator degrees of freedom. They correspond to the degrees of freedom of SS_A and SS_w, respectively. In short:

$$F \overset{H_0}{\sim} F_{J-1, N-J}.$$

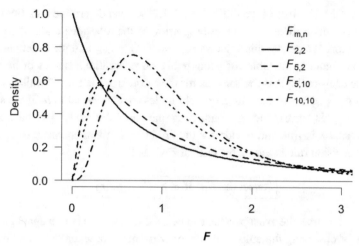

Fig. 8.4 Examples of probability density functions of different (central) F-distributions with m numerator and n denominator degrees of freedom

Figure 8.4 visualizes four different F-distributions. If a random variable X is F-distributed with m numerator and n denominator degrees of freedom, $X \sim F_{m,n}$, its expected value is $E(X) = \frac{n}{n-2}$ (for $n > 2$) and its variance is $\sigma_X^2 = \frac{2n^2(m+n-2)}{m(n-2)^2(n-4)}$ (for $n > 4$).

In Depth 8.2: The Relation Between F and t

With only two groups, we would normally compute a t-test for two independent samples, but we could also run an ANOVA just as well. This suggests that F and t might be related. Indeed, there is a direct relation that is valid only in case of two groups:

$$F = t^2. \tag{8.6}$$

In this case, the denominator degrees of freedom (i.e., df_w) are equal to the degrees of freedom of the corresponding t-distribution.

8.2.4 The Decision Rule

The F-ratio relates two expressions to each other: the numerator derives from the variability of the sample means, the denominator derives from the variability of the measured values within the groups. The resulting F-value becomes larger the more the data speak against the H_0. Just as we did in Sect. 5.1.2, we can determine a **critical F-value**, to the right of which there is a certain proportion of the total area under the probability density function. We denote this value as $F_{crit} = F_{J-1,N-J;\alpha}$ and the exact values of this cutoff can be found in the tables of many books on inferential statistics or be calculated with R. The decision logic is the same as for the t-test: If H_0 is true, F-values larger than or equal to $F_{J-1,N-J;\alpha}$ occur with a probability less than or equal to α. If we still obtain such a value—this corresponds to conducting one particular study—we have reasons to doubt that the H_0 is true and decide for the H_1 instead. We then speak of a significant result. The decision rule based on the critical F-value thus is:

$$\text{Reject the } H_0, \text{ if } F \geq F_{J-1,N-J;\alpha}.$$

In addition, of course, the exact p-value can be used for the decision: p again indicates the probability of observing the empirical or more extreme data when the H_0 is true. If it is less than or equal to α, we decide in favor of the H_1, because we question the assumption of H_0 being true. As before, both decision rules are equivalent:

$$F_{empirical} \geq F_{crit} \Leftrightarrow p \leq \alpha.$$

If we perform the test with $\alpha = 0.05$, the critical value for our example is $F_{crit} = 3.35$. Because $F = 12.07 \geq 3.35$, we decide in favor of the H_1. A calculation of the exact p-value results in $p = .00018$, and because $p \leq \alpha$, the decision is the same.

8.3   Effect Sizes and Power

We have introduced the concepts of effect size and power in Chap. 7 using the example of the t-tests. Similar considerations, of course, apply to the ANOVA as well. However, we can no longer use simple differences to quantify effects if we have three or more groups. We will therefore begin with discussing what is actually meant by an effect in ANOVA. This concept will then allow to estimate effects and compute statistical power.

8.3.1   Effect Sizes in the Population

The effect size δ was introduced in Sect. 7.2 for the comparison of two means. Obviously, we cannot use this measure with more than two groups, because in this case, we can no longer compute a simple difference between means. Therefore, we choose another approach.

If we consider all populations together, we can specify a common population mean, μ, which we call here the expected value of the grand mean. With Formula 8.3 we mentioned that the grand mean M of the data can also be understood as a weighted average of the group means M_j. A random variable M which assigns each combination of samples the grand mean M, moreover, has μ as the expected value. Hence, μ can also be written as a weighted average of the expected values μ_j of each population:

$$E(M) = \mu = \sum_{j=1}^{J} \frac{n_j}{N} \mu_j.$$

Now, each μ_j deviates from the grand expected value μ in a certain way, and we refer to this deviation as the *effect of level j of the factor* (on the dependent variable). The notation for this is usually α_j:[4]

$$\alpha_j = \mu_j - \mu \qquad \forall j \in \{1, \ldots, J\}. \tag{8.7}$$

In this way, there are exactly as many effects α_j as there are populations or groups. These effects always sum up to 0, and we therefore combine them into an effect *variance* σ_α^2:

$$\sigma_\alpha^2 = \sum_{j=1}^{J} \frac{n_j}{N} \underbrace{(\mu_j - \mu)^2}_{=\alpha_j}.$$

The closer this value is to 0, the more similar are the effects of the individual populations. Therefore, the H_0 of the ANOVA can also be written as $H_0 : \sigma_\alpha^2 = 0$.

Similar to the effect size δ (Formula 7.1), σ_α^2 is divided by the error variance σ^2, and the result is the effect size f^2:

$$f^2 = \frac{\sigma_\alpha^2}{\sigma^2}.$$

Another measure of effect size in the context of ANOVA is η^2 (a lowercase eta):[5]

$$\eta^2 = \frac{\sigma_\alpha^2}{\sigma_\alpha^2 + \sigma^2} = \frac{\sigma_\alpha^2}{\sigma_{\text{tot}}^2}.$$

---

[4] The use of the same Greek letter for multiple concepts is commonplace in statistics, and can be confusing at times. The just introduced α_j, for example, should not be confused with the probability of a Type I error . Also, there will be further uses for β in the following chapters, but the context should always allow for a correct interpretation.

[5] Instead of η^2, this quantity sometimes is also called ω^2.

The effect size η^2 can be interpreted as the proportion of the total variance explained by the effect variance σ_α^2. Moreover, both of these effect sizes can easily be converted into each other:

$$\eta^2 = \frac{f^2}{1 + f^2} \qquad \text{and} \qquad f^2 = \frac{\eta^2}{1 - \eta^2}.$$

To assess the size of such effects, Cohen (1988) proposed conventions for the effect size f (i.e., the square root of f^2). According to them, small, medium, and large effects are $f = 0.10$, $f = 0.25$, and $f = 0.40$, respectively. Expressed as η^2, this corresponds to $\eta^2 = 0.01$, $\eta^2 = 0.06$, and $\eta^2 = 0.14$, respectively.

8.3.2   Estimating the Effect Size from Samples

In the previous section, we considered how effect sizes are conceptualized in ANOVA. Because we had only considered such effect sizes at the population level—that is, as parameters—the next question is how to estimate them. The most frequently used measure of effect size in this context is η^2, and two variants exist for its estimation:

- The effect variance is estimated with SS_A and the total variance (i.e., here the sum of the effect variance and the error variance) is estimated with SS_{tot}. The complete estimator is then:

$$\hat{\eta}^2 = \frac{SS_A}{SS_{\text{tot}}}. \tag{8.8}$$

With the values we calculated in Sect. 8.2.1, the estimated effect size for our example is:

$$\hat{\eta}^2 = \frac{125.07}{264.97} = 0.47.$$

This value corresponds to the output of SPSS and the R package ez.[6] However, it systematically overestimates the population effect so that, for example, positive values result for $\hat{\eta}^2$ even for a population effect of $\eta^2 = 0$.

---

[6] Even though the outputs of both programs list the effect size as η^2, strictly speaking, we are looking at the corresponding estimator $\hat{\eta}^2$. When reporting this effect size, however, it has become common to speak of η^2.

- A different formula is sometimes used to estimate η^2 to counter the overestimation bias, even though this variant is not an unbiased estimator for η^2 either (instead of $\hat{\eta}^2$, it is sometimes called $\hat{\omega}^2$; see also Mordkoff 2019):

$$\hat{\eta}^2 = \frac{SS_A - (J - 1)MS_w}{SS_{\text{tot}} + MS_w}.$$

For the example data from this chapter, it yields an estimated effect of:

$$\hat{\eta}^2 = \frac{125.07 - 2 \cdot 5.18}{264.97 + 5.18} = 0.42.$$

8.3.3 Power of ANOVA

In Sect. 7.3, we introduced the concept of power: The probability of obtaining a significant result when a certain effect is present in the population. In this context, we had further introduced the non-central t-distribution. Now we apply these considerations to ANOVA and the F-distribution. So far, we have noted that the F-ratio follows a central F-distribution, assuming that the H_0 is true. However, if there is an effect in the population, the F-ratio follows a non-central F-distribution.

We have illustrated these situations for an F-distribution with $m = 6$ numerator and $n = 100$ denominator degrees of freedom in Fig. 8.5. With $\alpha = 0.05$, we would get a critical F-value of 2.19. The red area in the left panel of Fig. 8.5 cuts off the corresponding 5% of the area under the central F-distribution. Larger empirical F-values are possible under the assumption that the H_0 is true, while obtaining such results provides sufficient reasons to question the assumption of H_0. The right panel of Fig. 8.5 shows a non-central F-distribution (with a non-centrality parameter $\Delta = 20$). This is what the distribution of a corresponding random variable would look like if we drew the samples from populations for which a corresponding effect exists. Then, the area under this probability density function to the right of the critical F-value (i.e., the blue area) is the probability of obtaining a larger empirical F-value than the critical F-value, that is, the power $1 - \beta$. The orange area, on the other hand, corresponds to the probability of obtaining a non-significant result when this particular H_1 is true, thus the probability of committing a Type II error.

These interpretations are completely analogous to those in Sect. 7.3 for the t-distribution. This showcases how similar the procedures of null hypothesis significance testing are across individual significance tests.

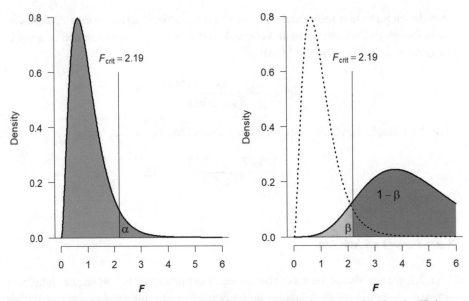

Fig. 8.5 The left panel visualizes a central F-distribution under the assumption that the H_0 is true, and the right panel additionally shows a non-central F-distribution under the assumption that a particular H_1 is true (with a non-centrality parameter $\Delta = 20$). In both panels, the distributions have $m = 6$ numerator and $n = 100$ denominator degrees of freedom

8.4   Contrasts in ANOVA

So far, we have tested global null hypotheses in the context of ANOVA; this is sometimes also called an *omnibus* ANOVA. In case of a significant result, however, all we know is that at least two of the population means are likely to differ. What we do not know is which of the means are actually different from one another. Such and even further questions can be answered by testing **contrasts**. Conceptually, there are two types of contrasts:

- Having obtained a significant result in an ANOVA, contrasts are often calculated to locate significant pairwise differences. These are so-called *a posteriori-contrasts*: They can only be tested in a non-directional way and may even not really be considered hypothesis tests at all, since no hypotheses about individual population means have been formulated in advance. For such purposes, there are various procedures, for example, the Scheffé test (Scheffé 1963), all of which include an α-adjustment by design, but differ in exactly how they implement the correction.
- We can specify and test (only) theoretically interesting contrasts a priori, that is, when hypotheses are based on specific predictions. These are so-called *a priori-contrasts* ("planned comparisons"). These contrasts are based on a design suited for an ANOVA, but ideally are even conducted instead of an omnibus ANOVA. In general, they are

preferable to a posteriori contrasts, because their hypotheses are typically based on theoretical considerations.

8.4.1 Examples of Contrasts

To get a grip on the different ways to formulate contrasts, we return to our introductory example in which participants completed a memory test after zero, 1, or 2 day(s) of sleep deprivation. The means of the data from Table 8.2 in these three conditions were 18.1, 15.7, and 13.1 words, so performance on the memory test decreases with increasing sleep deprivation, and the ANOVA was significant. Below we describe three scenarios that might be of interest in this example and that can indeed be analyzed with contrasts. With μ_1, μ_2, and μ_3 we denote the means of the populations from which the samples of the three factor levels are drawn:

- **Example 1:** A simple case would be to ask whether performance deteriorates already after just 1 day of sleep deprivation, that is, whether $\mu_1 > \mu_2$.

- **Example 2:** Perhaps there is reason to assume that performance would only drop after 2 days of sleep deprivation, while only 1 day of sleep deprivation leads to the same performance as without sleep deprivation. Such a prediction could be tested with two contrasts: The first contrast states that $\frac{\mu_1+\mu_2}{2} > \mu_3$, and the second contrast states that $\mu_1 = \mu_2$.

- **Example 3:** The factor levels in our example involve a natural order: One day of sleep deprivation is more than no day of sleep deprivation, 2 days of sleep deprivation are more than just 1 day of sleep deprivation, and these two differences are equal. This also allows testing the conjecture that performance on the memory test decreases linearly with the number of days of sleep deprivation. In this case, then, the difference on the dependent variable between each two of the adjacent factor levels should also be identical, so that $\mu_1 - \mu_2 = \mu_2 - \mu_3$.

What actually is a contrast? In technical terms, a contrast is nothing else than a certain combination of population parameters. We call this (linear) combination ψ (a lowercase psi), and we construct it by multiplying all μ_j with a coefficient c_j and then summing them up:

$$\psi = c_1\mu_1 + \ldots + c_J\mu_J = \sum_{j=1}^{J} c_j\mu_j. \tag{8.9}$$

It is important to note, however, that we only speak of a contrast when the c_j add up to 0 in total, that is, when:

$$\sum_{j=1}^{J} c_j = 0.$$

8.4.2   Hypotheses and Estimating Contrasts

We first consider the hypothesis pair of a contrast analysis and then explain its calculation. In all the following steps, the same assumptions apply as in the ANOVA (see Formula 8.2).

The hypothesis pair to be tested is usually identical for all contrasts: ψ is tested against the value 0. Thus, when the test is non-directional, the hypothesis pair is:

$$H_0: \quad \psi = 0 \qquad \text{and} \qquad H_1: \quad \psi \neq 0.$$

The major challenge with contrasts is to transform substantive hypotheses into contrast hypotheses. This is done by specifying the coefficients c_j, and we explain this for the three introductory examples:

- **Example 1:** $H_0: \mu_1 = \mu_2$ can be rephrased as $\mu_1 - \mu_2 = 0$. Adding the coefficients, we can write:

$$\underbrace{1 \cdot \mu_1 + (-1) \cdot \mu_2 + 0 \cdot \mu_3}_{= \psi} = 0.$$

  The left part of this formula is a contrast ψ and the coefficients are $c_1 = 1$, $c_2 = -1$, and $c_3 = 0$.

- **Example 2:** This example involves two contrasts as mentioned above. The H_0 of the first contrast, $\frac{\mu_1 + \mu_2}{2} = \mu_3$, can also be written as $\frac{\mu_1 + \mu_2}{2} - \mu_3 = 0$ and the coefficients are thus $c_1 = \frac{1}{2}$, $c_2 = \frac{1}{2}$, and $c_3 = -1$. The H_0 of the second contrast corresponds to that of Example 1.

- **Example 3:** Finally, the H_0 of this example, $\mu_1 - \mu_2 = \mu_2 - \mu_3$, can be written as $\mu_1 - 2\mu_2 + \mu_3 = 0$, and the coefficients are $c_1 = 1$, $c_2 = -2$, and $c_3 = 1$. Here we note that linearity is present in case the H_0 is true, and we should therefore be interested in a small probability of committing a Type II error.

Obviously, all μ_j can be estimated in each case with the corresponding mean M_j. Accordingly, a suitable estimator for the full contrast would be $\hat{\psi} = \sum_{j=1}^{J} c_j M_j$. Let us now consider a random variable $\hat{\psi}$ which assigns the estimator $\hat{\psi}$ to each combination of samples from the population(s) under consideration. Then, its expected value and variance are:

$$E(\hat{\psi}) = \psi \quad \text{and} \quad V(\hat{\psi}) = \sigma^2 \sum_{j=1}^{J} \frac{c_j^2}{n_j}.$$

Because $\hat{\psi}$ consists of a weighted sum of the normally distributed random variables M_j it is normally distributed as well:

$$\hat{\psi} \sim N(\psi, \sigma^2 \sum_{j=1}^{J} \frac{c_j^2}{n_j}).$$

Finally, we use

$$S_{\hat{\psi}}^2 = MS_w \sum_{j=1}^{J} \frac{c_j^2}{n_j},$$

as an unbiased estimator for $V(\hat{\psi})$, where MS_w is the mean sum of square that we had already encountered in the omnibus ANOVA.

8.4.3 Testing Contrast Hypotheses

How can we now use this information to test contrast hypotheses? The procedure is again identical to the procedure for t-tests and the ANOVA presented above: We construct a test statistic that involves $\hat{\psi}$ and that satisfies the two known conditions: (1) Its value becomes more extreme the more the data speak against the H_0 and (2) we can determine the distribution of a corresponding random variable assuming that the H_0 is true.

We have already considered the general form of the t-ratio in Formula 5.5. Applied to contrasts, this formula can be specified as:

$$t = \frac{T - \tau_0}{SE_T} = \frac{\hat{\psi} - 0}{\sqrt{S_{\hat{\psi}}^2}} = \frac{\hat{\psi}}{\sqrt{MS_w \sum_{j=1}^{J} \frac{c_j^2}{n_j}}}. \tag{8.10}$$

With this latter formula, we can calculate a particular empirical value from our data and we can also determine the distribution of this t-ratio: $t \overset{H_0}{\sim} t_{N-J}$ where N denotes the total number of participants and J denotes the number of factor levels. The decision rule in the non-directional case is thus:

$$\boxed{\text{Reject the } H_0, \text{ if } |t| \geq t_{N-J;\frac{\alpha}{2}} \text{ or if } p \leq \alpha.}$$

Because the denominator in Formula 8.10 uses MS_w, it uses information from all participants to estimate the population variance, and the denominator is usually smaller and the t-value is thus larger compared to the case of a simple t-test. Moreover, it relies on a t-distribution with more degrees of freedom, which results in smaller critical t-values. In summary, the power of contrasts is generally higher than that of the corresponding t-tests.

8.5   Concluding Remarks

8.5.1   Reporting ANOVA Results

In Sect. 8.2.4 we obtained a significant result for the ANOVA on the example data, but did not discuss the meaning of this result yet. For interpreting this outcome, we have to keep in mind that the H_1 only says that at least two of the involved μs are not identical; it does *not* state that all μs are different from each other. Accordingly, our significant result only means that at least two of the groups probably come from populations with different means. We do not know which these are—this would require the calculation of contrasts (see Sect. 8.4).

A detailed presentation of the results from an ANOVA is usually given in a table. For our example, Table 8.3 shows the complete results. If we wanted to report these results in articles or theses, for example, this could be done in the following way:

> The mean number of recalled words is shown in Fig. 8.1. The one-way ANOVA revealed a significant effect of sleep deprivation, $F(2, 27) = 12.07$, $p < .001$, $\eta^2 = .47$.

8.5.2   Confidence Intervals

For (two) independent samples, we have distinguished confidence intervals for the individual means (each based on the group's own variance) from a confidence interval for the mean difference (see Chap. 6).

Table 8.3 Full presentation of the results of a one-way ANOVA

Source of variance	df	SS	MS	F	p
Effect A (sleep deprivation)	2	125.07	62.53	12.07	< .001
Within (residual/error)	27	139.90	5.18		

With more than two groups, we can of course also compute a confidence interval for each individual group. The resulting confidence intervals provide information on whether the respective group mean differs significantly from a hypothetical population parameter (see also Sect. 6.3.1). These confidence intervals can also be informative for judging whether the assumption of homogeneity of variance is justified.

Most of the time, however, the focus will not be on deviations of individual group means from parameter values, but rather on differences between the means of different populations. In addition, we have made the assumption in Formula 8.2 that all groups come from populations with identical variance. If we are willing to accept this assumption to hold in our data, then this suggests to estimate the population variance on a common basis including all data. Indeed, we already know this common estimator: MS_w (Loftus and Masson 1994). This estimator is often more accurate (and smaller) than estimation based on a single sample variance. Moreover, MS_w has more degrees of freedom, and the t-value used as the certainty parameter is therefore smaller. Let us denote with N the total sample size and with J the number of factor levels. Then we can construct a confidence intervals as:

$$\left[M_j \pm t_{N-J;\frac{\alpha}{2}} \cdot \sqrt{\frac{MS_w}{n_j}} \right].$$

It is reasonable to assume that two group means are significantly different from each other in an appropriate contrast if one of those means is not included in the confidence interval around the other mean. In Sect. 6.4 (footnote 1) we have already referred to the factor $\sqrt{2}$, and we must take this factor into account if we want to estimate the standard error with MS_w from the ANOVA. At least in case of equal sample sizes, two means are significantly different if one mean is not in the confidence interval multiplied by the factor $\sqrt{2}$ around the other mean (see also Loftus and Masson 1994). In other words, two means M_k and M_m differ significantly if

$$|M_k - M_m| > \sqrt{2} \cdot t_{N-J;\frac{\alpha}{2}} \cdot \sqrt{\frac{MS_w}{n}} \qquad k, m \in \{1, \ldots, J\}.$$

8.5.3   Violated Assumptions

The correct derivation of the distribution of the F-ratio is subject to certain assumptions, which are summarized in Formula 8.2. Just as with the t-test, violations of these assumptions affect the validity of the result of an ANOVA.

Fortunately, the ANOVA is generally quite robust with regard to violations of the assumed *normal distribution*, in particular with sufficiently large sample sizes of $n_j > 25$. In case of strong violations, data can be normalized with appropriate transformations or non-parametric tests can serve as an alternative. The non-parametric equivalent of the

ANOVA presented here is the Kruskal-Wallis test (see, e.g., Bortz and Schuster 2010 or Keppel and Wickens 2004). This test can also be used when the dependent variable does not meet the level of an interval scale.

ANOVA is more vulnerable to violations of the assumption of *homogeneity of variance* (e.g., Wilcox 1987), which in turn can cause the test to behave liberally. This problem occurs especially when sample sizes differ across groups (Box 1954). Thus, studies should be planned with equal sample sizes whenever possible. A more comprehensive account of procedures for dealing with violations of assumptions can be found, for example, in Keppel and Wickens (2004).

8.5.4   Another Perspective on the One-Way ANOVA

In this last section, we want to explain ANOVA from a different angle, one that will help us understand certain concepts in the next chapter.

Let us consider each individual observation y_{ij}. Then, in each of the samples under consideration, there are n_j independent realizations y_{ij} of the random variable Y_j. If we construe these realizations as random variables as well, then, the assumption made in Formula 8.2 implies:

$$y_{ij} \sim N(\mu_j, \sigma^2) \qquad \forall j \in \{1, \dots, J\}, \forall i \in \{1, \dots, n_j\}. \tag{8.11}$$

Now we distinguish two types of deviations:

- We have introduced the deviation of an expected value μ_j from the grand expected value μ as the effect α_j in Sect. 8.3.1 (see Formula 8.7). This deviation is often called the *explained deviation*.
- In addition, each data point (i.e., participant) still deviates from the expected value of its group, that is, from μ_j. We can label this deviation as the *measurement error* e_{ij}. The deviation of participant i of sample j from the (group) parameter μ_j is therefore:

$$e_{ij} = y_{ij} - \mu_j. \tag{8.12}$$

Instead of measurement error, this deviation is also often called the *unexplained deviation*. Formula 8.11 further implies:

$$e_{ij} \sim N(0, \sigma^2).$$

The measurement error e_{ij} can therefore be regarded as a normally distributed random variable with an expected value of 0 and the same variance as the one we have *assumed* for the dependent variable.

Drawing on Formulas 8.7 and 8.12, we can now write every single value y_{ij} as:

$$y_{ij} = \mu + \alpha_j + e_{ij}. \tag{8.13}$$

In other words: Each value y_{ij} is composed additively of the grand expected value μ, the effect α_j of the respective factor level, and a measurement error e_{ij}. Formula 8.13 is also referred to as the **statistical model of the one-way ANOVA** (on the *level of empirical samples*).

If we are interested in the *statistical model on the level of population parameters*, we consider the expected values on both sides of Formula 8.13: We already know from the assumption made above (Formula 8.11) that the expected value of y_{ij} equals μ_j. Further, μ and α_j are constants, and the expected value of e_{ij} is 0. It thus follows that μ_j is composed additively of the grand expected value μ and the respective effect α_j:

$$\mu_j = \mu + \alpha_j. \tag{8.14}$$

We will return to Formula 8.14 in the next chapter.

8.6 Examples and Exercises

8.6.1 One-Way ANOVA with R

We now analyze the data from Table 8.2 with R. The underlying research question was: Does the amount of recalled words differ as a function of sleep deprivation?

The sample data from Table 8.2 are available in the online material in the file 8_data_ANOVA_sleep_deprivation.dat. It can be read with the function read.table() into a data frame named data. This data frame then comprises four variables: subject, sleep_deprivation, age, and recalled_words. To calculate the ANOVA, the variable sleep_deprivation must first be factorized. Factorizing provides attributes that are necessary for further use. This is especially true for the attribute level, which lists the individual levels of the factor:

```
data$sleep_deprivation <- as.factor(data$sleep_deprivation)
```

We can now compute the ANOVA. A general function for this is aov(), which requires at least two arguments. The first argument uses the modeling language of R and determines which dependent variable (recalled_words) is to be modeled by which factor(s) (sleep_deprivation). For our example, we thus use recalled_words ~ sleep_deprivation. As the second argument, we pass the data frame containing the factorized variables to the function:

```
aov_result <- aov(recalled_words ~ sleep_deprivation,
                  data = data)
```

The result of the ANOVA can be output with the function summary():

```
summary(aov_result)
                  Df Sum Sq Mean Sq F value   Pr(>F)
sleep_deprivation  2 125.07  62.533  12.069 0.0001801 ***
Residuals         27 139.90   5.181
```

The first line contains statistics for the factor sleep_deprivation (degrees of freedom, SS_A, MS_A), as well as the F-value and the corresponding p-value. The second line describes the error term with its degrees of freedom, SS_w, and MS_w. As expected, the calculation leads to the same result as the calculation by hand (Sect. 8.2.3): There is a significant effect of sleep deprivation, $F(2, 27) = 12.07$, $p < .001$. The calculation of η^2 is described in the online material.

In the one-way case, the modeling notation of the ANOVA is straightforward. For factorial ANOVA (Chap. 9) and ANOVA with repeated-measures (Chap. 10), using the function aov() becomes more complicated. Thus, we consider here an additional function that can be adapted very flexibly to many types of ANOVA and is included in the package ez. Once installed, this package needs to be loaded before use with library(ez).

The corresponding function ezANOVA() also requires the variable subject to be factorized. Then, the ANOVA is calculated with ezANOVA() requiring only a specification of the individual variables in the experimental design:

```
# factorize subject first
data$subject <- as.factor(data$subject)
ez_result <- ezANOVA(data = data,
                     wid = .(subject),
                     dv = .(recalled_words),
                     between = .(sleep_deprivation),
                     detailed = TRUE)
ez_result

$ANOVA
             Effect DFn DFd      SSn   SSd      F...
1 sleep_deprivation   2  27 125.0667 139.9 12.06862...
                              ...p p<.05          ges
                   ...0.0001800766     * 0.4720091

$'Levene's Test for Homogeneity of Variance'
  DFn DFd      SSn  SSd       F         p p<.05
1   2  27 7.466667 53.5 1.884112 0.1714068
```

The output corresponds to that of `summary(aov)`, but an estimator of an effect size is also directly calculated (column `ges`),[7] so we can report the full result, $F(2, 27) = 12.07$, $p < .001$, $\eta^2 = .47$. We can also obtain the formatted statistics with the function `anova_out()` of the package `schoRsch`. This function also provides an estimator for η_p^2 in its output:

```
anova_out(ez_result)

$`--- FORMATTED RESULTS ---------------------------------------------`
              Effect                                        Text
1 sleep_deprivation F(2,27) = 12.07, p < .001, np2 = .47
```

Note that the current version of `anova_out()` can only handle the output of `ezANOVA()`. Further details on specifying contrasts in R can be found in the online material for this chapter.

8.6.2 One-Way ANOVA with SPSS

We now analyze the data from Table 8.2 with SPSS. The underlying research question was: Does the amount of recalled words differ as a function of sleep deprivation?

The file `8_data_ANOVA_sleep_deprivation.sav` provides the sample data. There are two ways for calculating a one-way ANOVA with SPSS. The first one is accessed via the menu

```
Analyze > Compare Means > One-Way ANOVA...
```

This menu opens a dialog box (Fig. 8.6), in which we move the dependent variable (`Recalled_Words`) and the factor (`Sleep_Deprivation`) into the corresponding fields. Clicking on *Options* allows for requesting additional statistics as well as a figure of the means. The output (Fig. 8.7) provides the descriptive statistics (if requested) as well as a table that (by and large) corresponds to the previously presented Table 8.3. It summarizes the sums of squares, the degrees of freedom, the F-value, and the corresponding p-value. For our example, there is a significant effect of sleep deprivation, $F(2, 27) = 12.07$, $p < .001$.

---

[7] This effect size is called *generalized* η^2 (Olejnik and Algina 2003). In many cases, it corresponds to η^2 (or η_p^2, which we will introduce in Chap. 9). However, there are cases where the two values do not correspond. In the online material, we describe how to determine η^2 or η_p^2 from the result of `ezANOVA()`.

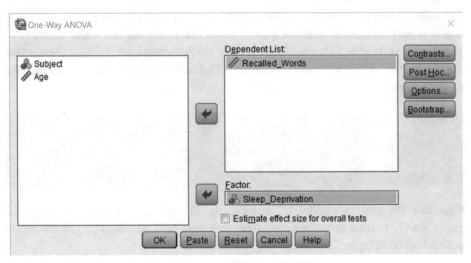

Fig. 8.6   Dialog box for conducting a one-way ANOVA with SPSS

Descriptives

Recalled_Words

	N	Mean	Std. Deviation	Std. Error	95% Confidence Interval for Mean		Minimum	Maximum
					Lower Bound	Upper Bound		
0	10	18.10	2.183	.690	16.54	19.66	14	22
1	10	15.70	1.494	.473	14.63	16.77	13	18
2	10	13.10	2.923	.924	11.01	15.19	8	17
Total	30	15.63	3.023	.552	14.50	16.76	8	22

ANOVA

Recalled_Words

	Sum of Squares	df	Mean Square	F	Sig.
Between Groups	125.067	2	62.533	12.069	.000
Within Groups	139.900	27	5.181		
Total	264.967	29			

Fig. 8.7   SPSS output for a one-way ANOVA

A drawback of this method is that it cannot directly provide an estimator of an effect size and it is also limited to a single factor. A more general variant for carrying out an ANOVA can be accessed via the menu

```
Analyze > General Linear Model > Univariate...
```

In the following dialog box (Fig. 8.8, left panel), we move the dependent variable (recalled_words) into the corresponding field, and the (single) factor (sleep_deprivation) into the field *Fixed Factor(s)*. Further options can be accessed

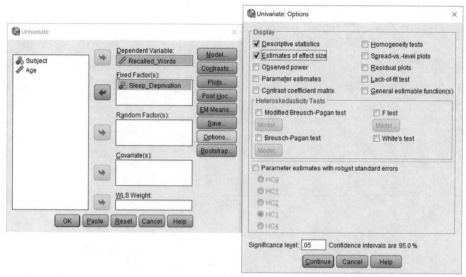

Fig. 8.8 Dialog boxes for performing an ANOVA with SPSS in the context of the general linear model. The left panel shows the dialog box for specifying dependent variable and factor(s), the right panel shows the *Options* dialog box, which can also be used to request an effect size estimator

by clicking on *Options* (Fig. 8.8, right panel). With this dialog box, in addition to descriptive statistics, we can also request effect size estimators and should therefore tick the corresponding box. A visualization can be requested with the field *Plots*. Clicking on *OK* opens the output window with all requested information. Inferential statistics are provided in the table *Tests of Between-Subjects Effects*. In the present example, there is a significant effect of sleep deprivation, $F(2, 27) = 12.07, p < .001, \eta^2 = .47$. The degrees of freedom can be obtained from the lines *Sleep_Deprivation* and *Error*.

SPSS provides several predefined contrasts, which are described in the Command Syntax Reference. This applies to all types of ANOVA within the General Linear Model that can be performed via the menu items *Univariate* and *Repeated Measures*. Furthermore, the syntax of these ANOVAs can be extended to specify custom contrasts. For example, the comparison of 2 days of sleep deprivation with no day of sleep deprivation can be requested using the equivalent commands

```
/CONTRAST(Sleep_Deprivation) = SPECIAL(1,0,-1)
```

and

```
/LMATRIX = '2 vs. 0', Sleep_Deprivation 1 0 -1
```

Contrasts are always tested with the *F*-distribution in SPSS. However, the results can easily be converted to a *t*-value if necessary (see Formula 8.6).

Factorial Analysis of Variance (ANOVA)

9

Many empirical studies involve two or more independent variables. Analysis of variance (ANOVA) can easily be extended to these situations. To this end, we extend the one-way (or single-factor) ANOVA to multiple factors in this chapter. To understand the general idea of factorial ANOVA, we start by considering the two-factor (or two-way) ANOVA, before briefly addressing the case of three (or more) factors at the end of the chapter. The concept of factorial ANOVA is also required for understanding ANOVA with repeated measures (Chap. 10).

When introducing the one-way ANOVA, we considered the influence of sleep deprivation on memory performance as an example. Briefly, performance deteriorated with increasing sleep deprivation and the ANOVA yielded a significant result. Now, a critical reader of our results might highlight that there is evidence for this effect to depend on age and that we did not adequately account for the age of the participants in our analysis. More precisely, the (new) hypothesis states that memory performance would only decline in older, but not in younger adults.

We therefore split the sample (Table 8.2) within each level of the factor "sleep deprivation" into "younger adults" (under 40 years of age) and "older adults" (40 years and older). The resulting data are summarized in Table 9.1. We can see from the descriptive data that memory performance indeed declines more rapidly in the older than in the younger participants.

The hypothesis formulated above could, in principle, be tested using separate one-way ANOVAs for younger and older adults each. Doing so would come with various issues, however. Similar to the comparison of multiple t-tests versus one-way ANOVA, these are loss of power, α-inflation, etc. Therefore, the analysis of choice in this case is a **two-way**

© Springer-Verlag GmbH Germany, part of Springer Nature 2023
M. Janczyk, R. Pfister, *Understanding Inferential Statistics*,
https://doi.org/10.1007/978-3-662-66786-6_9

Table 9.1 Sample data for a two-way ANOVA (based on Table 8.2)

	Younger adults (<40 yrs.)			Older adults (≥40 yrs.)		
	Sleep deprivation			Sleep deprivation		
	0 days	1 day	2 days	0 days	1 day	2 days
	22	18	17	17	15	12
	19	16	16	18	15	11
	18	16	15	16	14	10
	14	17	13	19	16	8
	18	17	16	20	13	13
M	18.2	16.8	15.4	18.0	14.6	10.8
S^2	6.56	0.56	1.84	2.00	1.04	2.96

ANOVA with the factors "sleep deprivation" (three levels) and "age group" (two levels). We will use this example to work through the basics of two-way ANOVA and later consider the general case beyond this example.

9.1   Basics of the Two-Way ANOVA

Our example comprises six different combinations of age group and days of sleep deprivation. The combinations are again associated with the respective populations, which can differ with respect to the parameter μ_{jk} (cf. Table 9.2). The index j denotes the level of the first factor "sleep deprivation", the index k denotes the level of the second factor "age group". The variance σ^2 is again assumed to be identical in all populations. Hence, it follows for the dependent variable Y_{jk}:

$$Y_{jk} \sim N(\mu_{jk}, \sigma^2) \qquad \forall j \in \{1, 2, 3\}, \forall k \in \{1, 2\}.$$

As for the one-way ANOVA, further assumptions are an interval-scaled dependent variable and independent samples. An additional restriction here is that all samples should be of equal size. This makes the approach to ANOVA considered here computationally simpler.

Table 9.2 The six combinations of sleep deprivation and age group from the example data with corresponding expected values μ_{jk} as well as the expected marginal means $\mu_{j.}$ and $\mu_{.k}$ and the global expected mean μ

		Factor A			
		(Sleep deprivation)			
		0 days	1 day	2 days	
Factor B	< 40	μ_{11}	μ_{21}	μ_{31}	$\mu_{.1}$
(Age group)	≥ 40	μ_{12}	μ_{22}	μ_{32}	$\mu_{.2}$
		$\mu_{1.}$	$\mu_{2.}$	$\mu_{3.}$	μ

Computer programs do not need this restriction, but it is still advisable to plan with equal sample sizes (details on this can be found in Box 9.2).

The so-called *marginal expected means* $\mu_{j\cdot}$ and $\mu_{\cdot k}$ play an important role in the following argument, and these are calculated for each level of one factor across all levels of the other factor. The period replaces the index of the factor across which the average is calculated (Table 9.2). Thus, for the factor sleep deprivation of our example, the expected marginal means are calculated as

$$\mu_{1\cdot} = \frac{\mu_{11} + \mu_{12}}{2} \quad \text{and} \quad \mu_{2\cdot} = \frac{\mu_{21} + \mu_{22}}{2} \quad \text{and} \quad \mu_{3\cdot} = \frac{\mu_{31} + \mu_{32}}{2},$$

and for the factor age group they are calculated as

$$\mu_{\cdot 1} = \frac{\mu_{11} + \mu_{21} + \mu_{31}}{3} \quad \text{and} \quad \mu_{\cdot 2} = \frac{\mu_{12} + \mu_{22} + \mu_{32}}{3}.$$

9.1.1 Main Effects

We first focus on the so-called **main effects**. In the example, we could perform a one-way ANOVA with the factor sleep deprivation and disregard the factor age group. A second possibility would be to perform such an ANOVA with the factor age group, disregarding the factor sleep deprivation. A similar procedure is also used in the two-way ANOVA, but the power is increased by taking the other factor into account (see also Sect. 9.3.1). It is important to note that the main effects do not tell us anything about whether—in the context of our example—the effect of sleep deprivation differs between younger or older adults. Rather, main effects describe how sleep deprivation or age group generally (i.e., across all levels of the other factor) affect performance.

In the terminology of ANOVA, main effects test differences between the expected marginal means of the individual levels of each factor. There are always as many main effect hypotheses as there are factors. Very similar to the pair of hypotheses in one-way ANOVA, those are in our example:

- **Main effect A (sleep deprivation):**

$$H_0^A : \quad \mu_{1\cdot} = \mu_{2\cdot} = \mu_{3\cdot}$$
$$H_1^A : \quad \mu_{m\cdot} \neq \mu_{n\cdot} \text{ for at least one pair } m, n \in \{1, 2, 3\}$$

- **Main effect B (age group):**

$$H_0^B : \quad \mu_{\cdot 1} = \mu_{\cdot 2}$$
$$H_1^B : \quad \mu_{\cdot 1} \neq \mu_{\cdot 2}$$

Table 9.3 Specific μ_{jk} as well as the expected marginal means and the total expected mean. The upper part of the table contains the expected values predicted using the mean values of the example data set, the lower part the expected values predicted on the basis of a main effect model (Formula 9.2)

Expected values estimated from example data					
		Factor *A* (Sleep deprivation)			
		0 days	1 day	2 days	
Factor *B*	< 40 yrs.	18.20	16.80	15.40	16.80
(Age group)	≥ 40 yrs.	18.00	14.60	10.80	14.47
		18.10	15.70	13.10	15.63

Expected values predicted from the main effect model					
		Factor *A* (Sleep deprivation)			
		0 days	1 day	2 days	
Factor *B*	< 40 yrs.	19.27	16.87	14.27	16.80
(Age group)	≥ 40 yrs.	16.94	14.54	11.94	14.47
		18.10	15.70	13.10	15.63

As a next step, we introduce—analogously to the one-way ANOVA (Sect. 8.3.1)—*effects* and denote these effects of the two factors as α_j and β_k:

$$\alpha_j = \mu_{j\cdot} - \mu \quad \forall j \in \{1, 2, 3\} \quad \text{and} \quad \beta_k = \mu_{\cdot k} - \mu \quad \forall k \in \{1, 2\}. \tag{9.1}$$

Let us now (tentatively) assume that the empirical means (Table 9.1) correspond to the population means μ_{jk}. This case and the resulting expected marginal means are shown in the upper part of Table 9.3. From there, we can now calculate the respective effects by subtracting the grand expected mean from the expected marginal means (Eq. 9.1). The respective effects add up to 0 (with minor rounding errors in the following numbers at the chosen number of decimals):

$$\alpha_1 = 2.47 \quad \alpha_2 = 0.07 \quad \alpha_3 = -2.53 \quad \text{and} \quad \beta_1 = 1.17 \quad \beta_2 = -1.16.$$

We can now formulate a *preliminary* model equation with these effects α_j and β_k (just as in one-way ANOVA; see Eq. 8.14). The equation of this main effect model is:

$$\mu_{jk} = \mu + \alpha_j + \beta_k. \tag{9.2}$$

Now let us calculate the μ_{jk} using this formula (the results are shown in the lower part of Table 9.3) and compare them with the values in the upper part of that table. It becomes clear that the empirical values and the values predicted by Eq. 9.2 do *not* match. Thus, the main effect model does not adequately explain the data. Therefore, we will extend it in the following section and introduce so-called interaction effects.

9.1.2 Interaction Effects

The main effect model assumes *pure additivity*. This is the case when the expected values of each cell can actually be calculated as $\mu_{jk} = \mu + \alpha_j + \beta_k$: The expected value μ_{jk} of each cell is then additively composed of the grand expected value μ and the (involved) effects α_j and β_k. In general, however, this additivity does not hold, and we call the differences between the actual values and the values predicted by the main effect model **interactions** (of the factors A and B). We denote these interactions by $(\alpha\beta)_{jk}$ and calculate them as:

$$(\alpha\beta)_{jk} = \mu_{jk} - (\mu + \alpha_j + \beta_k) = \mu_{jk} - \mu - \alpha_j - \beta_k.$$

Interaction effects are thus nothing more than the (systematic) deviation from pure additivity of the main effects. In other words, if all interaction effects are $(\alpha\beta)_{jk} = 0$, then we have pure additivity. With the interaction effects we can now formulate a model equation that is always valid:

$$\mu_{jk} = \mu + \alpha_j + \beta_k + (\alpha\beta)_{jk}.$$

If we additionally denote the measurement error of a person i in the group representing the combination of the factor levels j and k with e_{ijk}, then each corresponding measured value is defined as:

$$y_{ijk} = \mu + \alpha_j + \beta_k + (\alpha\beta)_{jk} + e_{ijk}.$$

In addition to the two main effect hypotheses, the two-way ANOVA further includes an interaction hypothesis:

- **Interaction effect AB (sleep deprivation $\times$ age group):**

$$H_0^{AB}: \quad (\alpha\beta)_{jk} = 0 \quad \forall j \in \{1, 2, 3\}, \forall k \in \{1, 2\}$$
$$H_1^{AB}: \quad \text{there is at least one } (\alpha\beta)_{jk} \neq 0 \quad j \in \{1, 2, 3\}, k \in \{1, 2\}$$

Of course, we will rarely if ever find an empirical data set in which the interaction completely vanishes (i.e., becomes 0), even if this was true in the population. Just as with any other inferential statistical procedure, we assume the H_0 to test the interaction hypothesis and the question is: How likely are the observed or more extreme deviations under this assumption? If they are very unlikely, we doubt the assumption of the H_0 and assume that there is an interaction of both factors, that is, a deviation from pure additivity.

9.1.3 Interpretation and Graphical Representation

Graphically, a two-way ANOVA is often illustrated with grouped bar plots or with line plots as in Fig. 9.1 (upper panel). As usual, the dependent variable is plotted on the y-axis. One factor is then plotted on the x-axis, while separate lines are drawn for each level of the second factor.

The two lower panels of Fig. 9.1 additionally illustrate the main effects. For the main effect A, we average across the two levels of factor B. Thus, we would compare the three large gray dots indicating the means of both age groups under the respective levels of the factor sleep deprivation (Fig. 9.1, lower left panel): performance—averaged across both age groups—thus becomes worse with increasing sleep deprivation (this corresponds to the one-way ANOVA as introduced in Chap. 8). Similarly, the main effect B compares the large white dot and the large black dot, which are the means of the respective age groups

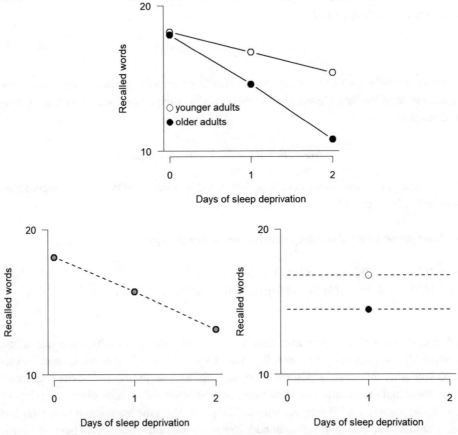

Fig. 9.1 The upper panel visualizes data that can be analyzed with a two-way ANOVA, and the lower panels illustrate the main effects

averaged across the days of sleep deprivation: the performance of the older adults is thus worse than that of younger adults (Fig. 9.1, lower right panel).

Note further that the lines for the two age groups in the upper panel of Fig. 9.1 are not parallel to each other. This signals the presence of an interaction. Conversely, if the lines representing the levels of a factor run parallel to each other, there is no interaction, but the factors combine additively.

An interaction thus means that the magnitude of the effect of one factor differs across the levels of the second factor. This becomes particularly clear in the upper panel of Fig. 9.1: Without sleep deprivation, the two age groups hardly differ in their performance, whereas with increasing sleep deprivation, we observe larger and larger differences. Let us now come back to the question from the beginning of this chapter. It should have become clear by now, that the two main effects do not say anything about differences of the effect of sleep deprivation between the two age groups. However, this question is addressed by testing the interaction of the two factors—and this is a major advantage of a two-way ANOVA over two one-way ANOVAs.

> **In Depth 9.1: Differences of Differences**
> Sometimes, scientific articles state that, for example, there was a certain significant effect for an experimental group, while this effect was not significant for the control group. Such a result is then interpreted as a difference in effect size *between* the two groups. Statistically, however, this statement is not necessarily correct (Cantor 1956; Nieuwenhuis et al. 2011): the difference in the size of a significant and a non-significant effect may itself *not* be statistically significant. A sound statement about any such difference requires a significant interaction between the factor of interest and the group factor.

9.2 Calculation

Having outlined the idea of two-way ANOVAs in our example, we now move on to its actual calculation. The procedure is conceptually identical to that of the one-way ANOVA: First, we quantify the total variability of the data with the total sum of squares SS_{tot} and decompose it into individual components. We convert these components into the mean sums of squares, and from these, we finally compute F-values, which we use to make decisions.[1]

---

[1] The individual computational steps using the example data can be found in the supplementary online material.

Table 9.4 The μ_{jk} of the combinations of two factors with J and K levels as well as the expected marginal means $\mu_{j\cdot}$ and $\mu_{\cdot k}$ and the grand expected mean μ

		\multicolumn{5}{c}{Factor A}			
		A_1	$\cdots$	A_j	$\cdots$	A_J	
	B_1	μ_{11}	$\cdots$	μ_{j1}	$\cdots$	μ_{J1}	$\mu_{\cdot 1}$
	$\vdots$	$\vdots$		$\vdots$		$\vdots$	$\vdots$
Factor B	B_k	μ_{1k}	$\cdots$	μ_{jk}	$\cdots$	mu_{Jk}	$\mu_{\cdot k}$
	$\vdots$	$\vdots$		$\vdots$		$\vdots$	$\vdots$
	B_K	μ_{1K}	$\cdots$	μ_{jK}	$\cdots$	μ_{JK}	$\mu_{\cdot K}$
		$\mu_{1\cdot}$	$\cdots$	$\mu_{j\cdot}$	$\cdots$	$\mu_{J\cdot}$	μ

In the general case, the factor A has J levels and the factor B has K levels. This results in a scheme of expected values as shown in Table 9.4. The expected marginal means are thus calculated as

$$\mu_{j\cdot} = \frac{1}{K} \sum_{k=1}^{K} \mu_{jk} \quad \forall j \in \{1, \dots, J\} \quad \text{and} \quad \mu_{\cdot k} = \frac{1}{J} \sum_{j=1}^{J} \mu_{jk} \quad \forall k \in \{1, \dots, K\},$$

and the grand expected mean μ is calculated as

$$\mu = \frac{1}{JK} \sum_{j=1}^{J} \sum_{k=1}^{K} \mu_{jk} \quad \text{or} \quad \mu = \frac{1}{J} \sum_{j=1}^{J} \mu_{j\cdot} = \frac{1}{K} \sum_{k=1}^{K} \mu_{\cdot k}.$$

The grand expected mean is thus either calculated as the mean of all expected values μ_{jk} or as the mean of the expected marginal means $\mu_{\cdot k}$ or $\mu_{j\cdot}$. The three hypotheses are:

- **Main effect A:**

  $H_0^A :\quad \mu_{1\cdot} = \mu_{2\cdot} = \dots = \mu_{J\cdot}$
  $H_1^A :\quad \mu_{m\cdot} \neq \mu_{n\cdot}$ for at least one pair $m, n \in \{1, \dots, J\}$

- **Main effect B:**

  $H_0^B :\quad \mu_{\cdot 1} = \mu_{\cdot 2} = \dots = \mu_{\cdot K}$
  $H_1^B :\quad \mu_{\cdot m} \neq \mu_{\cdot n}$ for at least one pair $m, n \in \{1, \dots, K\}$

- **Interaction effect AB:**

  $H_0^{AB} :\quad (\alpha\beta)_{jk} = 0 \quad \forall j \in \{1, \dots, J\}, \forall k \in \{1, \dots, K\}$
  $H_1^{AB} :\quad$ there is at least one $(\alpha\beta)_{jk} \neq 0 \quad j \in \{1, \dots, J\}, k \in \{1, \dots, K\}$

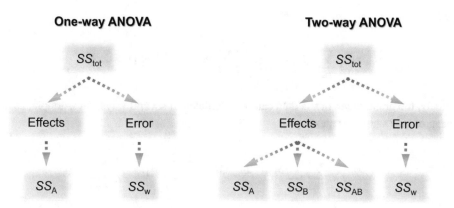

Fig. 9.2 Partitioning of sums of squares for one-way (left panel) and two-way (right panel) ANOVAs

9.2.1 Partitioning of Sums of Squares

In the context of one-way ANOVA, we had already encountered the concept of partitioning sums of squares: A kind of total variance, the SS_{tot}, was expressed as the sum of two other variance-like terms SS_A and SS_w. This is illustrated in the left panel of Fig. 9.2. We now apply this to the case of two-way ANOVA. However, here we can split SS_{tot} into a total of four components: those parts that are due to the main effects of both factors A and B (SS_A and SS_B, respectively), the part that is due to their interaction AB (SS_{AB}), and the part that is due to measurement error (SS_w). This partitioning is shown in the right panel of Fig. 9.2.

We now calculate these sums of squares in the following. With y_{ijk} we denote the measured value of a person i in that group that results from the combination of level j of the factor A and level k of the factor B. With sample size n, the means M_{jk} are then calculated as:

$$M_{jk} = \frac{1}{n} \sum_{i=1}^{n} y_{ijk} \qquad \forall j \in \{1, \ldots, J\}, \forall k \in \{1, \ldots, K\}.$$

Next, the marginal means of each factor level across the levels of the other factor are

$$M_{j\cdot} = \frac{1}{K} \sum_{k=1}^{K} M_{jk} = \frac{1}{nK} \sum_{k=1}^{K} \sum_{i=1}^{n} y_{ijk} \qquad \forall j \in \{1, \ldots, J\}$$

and

$$M_{\cdot k} = \frac{1}{J} \sum_{j=1}^{J} M_{jk} = \frac{1}{nJ} \sum_{j=1}^{J} \sum_{i=1}^{n} y_{ijk} \qquad \forall k \in \{1, \ldots, K\}.$$

Finally, the grand mean of the data can be calculated in several ways, for example, as the mean of the (marginal) means

$$M = \frac{1}{JK} \sum_{j=1}^{J} \sum_{k=1}^{K} M_{jk} \quad \text{or} \quad M = \frac{1}{J} \sum_{j=1}^{J} M_{j\cdot} = \frac{1}{K} \sum_{k=1}^{K} M_{\cdot k}$$

or directly from the raw data:

$$M = \frac{1}{nJK} \sum_{j=1}^{J} \sum_{k=1}^{K} \sum_{i=1}^{n} y_{ijk}.$$

These values are now used to calculate the corresponding sums of squares. These sums of squares also have certain degrees of freedom, which we directly specify here. In the following formulas, N denotes the total number of all data points, that is $N = nJK$:

$$SS_{\text{tot}} = \sum_{j=1}^{J} \sum_{k=1}^{K} \sum_{i=1}^{n} (y_{ijk} - M)^2 \quad \text{and} \quad df_{\text{tot}} = N - 1$$

$$SS_A = nK \sum_{j=1}^{J} (M_{j\cdot} - M)^2 \quad \text{and} \quad df_A = J - 1$$

$$SS_B = nJ \sum_{k=1}^{K} (M_{\cdot k} - M)^2 \quad \text{and} \quad df_B = K - 1$$

$$SS_{AB} = \sum_{j=1}^{J} \sum_{k=1}^{K} (M_{jk} - M_{j\cdot} - M_{\cdot k} + M)^2 \quad \text{and} \quad df_{AB} = (J - 1)(K - 1)$$

$$SS_w = \sum_{j=1}^{J} \sum_{k=1}^{K} \sum_{i=1}^{n} (y_{ijk} - M_{jk})^2 \quad \text{and} \quad df_w = JK(n - 1) = N - JK.$$

Just as in one-way ANOVA, the sums of squares of the effects and the sum of squares of the error (SS_w) add up to SS_{tot}:

$$SS_{\text{tot}} = SS_A + SS_B + SS_{AB} + SS_w.$$

9.2.2 Mean Sums of Squares

From the sums of squares as just calculated, we can now determine the corresponding mean sums of squares by dividing the sums of squares by their respective degrees of freedom. The mean sums of square of the three effects are:

$$MS_A = \frac{SS_A}{J-1}, \qquad MS_B = \frac{SS_B}{K-1}, \qquad \text{and} \qquad MS_{AB} = \frac{SS_{AB}}{(J-1)(K-1)},$$

and the mean sum of squares of the error term is:

$$MS_w = \frac{SS_w}{N-JK}.$$

9.2.3 F-Ratios and Decision Rules

In the final step—again exactly as in the one-way ANOVA—the mean sums of squares are used to calculate the corresponding F-ratios or F-values. More precisely, one F-value is calculated for each pair of hypotheses and the numerator of each F-ratio is the mean sum of squares of the relevant effect. The denominator is always MS_w, that is, we always use the same error term.

These F-values again fulfill exactly the two properties that we need for every test statistic: (1) They come with particularly extreme values the more the data speak against the H_0, and (2) their distribution is known under the assumption that the corresponding H_0 is true:

$$F^A = \frac{MS_A}{MS_w} \overset{H_0^A}{\sim} F_{J-1,N-JK}$$

$$F^B = \frac{MS_B}{MS_w} \overset{H_0^B}{\sim} F_{K-1,N-JK}$$

$$F^{AB} = \frac{MS_{AB}}{MS_w} \overset{H_0^{AB}}{\sim} F_{(J-1)(K-1),N-JK}.$$

Thus, the three test statistics are F-distributed, usually with different degrees of freedom. The decision rules for the three hypotheses, however, are analogous to the decision rule for the one-way ANOVA:

Reject the H_0, if $F \geq F_{\text{crit}}$ or if $p \leq \alpha$.

In Depth 9.2: Type I-III Sums of Squares

Our example data included samples of equal size. In such orthogonal designs, the sum of squares of one factor (e.g., sleep deprivation) is independent of whether the second factor (i.e., age group) is included in the analysis or not (here, we get $SS_A = 125.07$ either way; compare Tables 8.3 and 9.5). When sample sizes differ across the design cells of our analysis (i.e., when dealing with non-orthogonal designs), adding a factor changes the sum of squares of the other factor (Iacobucci 1995). Suppose we had studied not 5 younger and 5 older adults in the condition with 2 days of sleep deprivation, but 2 younger and 8 older adults instead. The low memory performance observed in Chap. 8 could then be due to both the effect of sleep deprivation or due to the larger proportion of older adults.

Different variants to calculate the sums of squares have been proposed to address such issues. They mainly differ in how they account for components of variability that can be equally attributed to both factors (as well as their interaction). *Type I* sums of squares are called hierarchical or sequential. Here, the sums of squares are initially calculated for one factor only (see Chap. 8; SS_A), to which these sums of squares attribute all parts of the variability this factor can explain (i.e., unique parts and those that are shared with other factors). The remaining unexplained variability is then used to calculate SS_B and, again, the remaining variability is used to calculate SS_{AB}. This leads to the useful property of additivity ($SS_{tot} = SS_A + SS_B + SS_{AB} + SS_w$), but the results eventually depend on the order of the factors. *Type II* sums of squares are called partially sequential, and they compute the sum of squares of each factor after attributing all shared variability to the other factor (i.e., SS_A is calculated on the variability that is not explained by factor B, and vice versa). Subsequently, SS_{AB} is calculated on the remaining variance. Type II sums of squares are calculated as the default, for example, in the functions of the R package ez. *Type III* sums of squares are the standard procedure of other statistical packages (including SPSS). They calculate the variability of individual effects only from those parts of the variability that can clearly be attributed to that factor and not to other factor(s) or interactions.

Type II or III sums of squares are generally recommended for unequal sample sizes. The former have a higher power for testing main effects, but these can only be interpreted in the absence of an interaction, since its effect is not controlled for when calculating SS_A and SS_B. The latter usually have less power, but the results can be interpreted in any case. With equal sample sizes across design cells, all methods produce identical results.

9.3   Concluding Remarks

9.3.1   Advantages of Factorial ANOVA

At the beginning of this chapter, we asked whether two one-way ANOVAs would be sufficient instead of a two-way ANOVA. Obviously, this is not the case, because only a factorial ANOVA allows to also examine the interplay of the factors, that is, their interaction.

Yet, there is another advantage of two main effect hypotheses over two one-way ANOVAs. Assume that a study has actually a two-factor design; however, we compute a one-way ANOVA only. Then, we get $SS_{tot} = SS_A + SS_w$, but the value of SS_A in the one-way ANOVA corresponds to SS_A in orthogonal two-way ANOVA. Thus, the effect of the first factor does not change when a second factor is taken into account (i.e., when calculating a two-way ANOVA). However, this also means that, in the case of one single factor, the error term SS_w actually comprises three different terms, whereas the two-way ANOVA removes variance from this term by estimating additional effects, namely $SS_B + SS_{AB} + SS_w$. Since SS_B and SS_{AB} are always larger than zero, it follows that SS_w is smaller in the two-way than in the one-way ANOVA. Because the error term is the denominator of the F-ratio, the F-value becomes larger the smaller the error term is. Any effect is thus more likely to be significant in a factorial ANOVA. This is often expressed by saying that parts of the total variability are attributed to the second factor or the interaction of both factors.

This can be seen when comparing Tables 8.3 and 9.5. In both cases, we get $SS_A = 125.07$. In addition, for the one-way ANOVA, the error term is $SS_w = 139.90$, and this value corresponds to the sum $SS_B + SS_{AB} + SS_w$ of the two-way ANOVA.

9.3.2   Effect Sizes

As an important measure of effect sizes in the context of ANOVAs, we had introduced the proportion of effect variance relative to the total variance (Chap. 8):

$$\eta^2 = \frac{\sigma_\alpha^2}{\sigma_{tot}^2}.$$

In case of multiple factors, the total variance is now composed of the variability attributed to all the effects involved plus the error variance. Therefore, a different measure is often used here, which is referred to as **partial** η^2. Here, the effect variance is no longer expressed as the proportion of the total variance, but of the sum of the relevant effect variance and the error variance:

$$\eta_p^2 = \frac{\sigma_{Effect}^2}{\sigma_{Effect}^2 + \sigma^2}.$$

Since the denominator for η_p^2 is smaller than for η^2, it follows that $\eta_p^2 > \eta^2$. For this reason, the sum of η_p^2 of all effects can also exceed 1; for η^2 this is not possible (cf. Pierce et al. 2004).

Similar to η^2 (see Sect. 8.3.2), η_p^2 can be estimated via the (mean) sums of squares. Most computer programs use the following formula:

$$\hat{\eta}_p^2 = \frac{SS_{\text{Effect}}}{SS_{\text{Effect}} + SS_w}.$$

Alternatively, a more conservative estimate can be used here as well:

$$\hat{\eta}_p^2 = \frac{SS_{\text{Effect}} - df_{\text{Effect}} \cdot MS_w}{SS_{\text{Effect}} + (N - df_{\text{Effect}}) \cdot MS_w}.$$

9.3.3   Interpretation and Presentation of Results

Factorial ANOVAs are typically best visualized in the form of line or bar plots (see Sect. 9.1.3). In order to interpret the (significant) results, they should also be presented in the text (see sect. 8.5.1) or as summarized in Table 9.5. As an alternative to the notation AB for the interaction, the notation $A \times B$ is frequently used.

Correctly interpreting the results is only possible by considering the descriptive means as well. Particularly in case of a significant interaction, the main effects should be interpreted cautiously: It is possible that a significant effect of one factor shows up only at certain levels of the other factor and is absent—or even reversed—at other levels.

9.3.4   ANOVA with More Than Two Factors

So far, we have considered only two factors, and a corresponding ANOVA already allows testing three pairs of hypotheses: main effect A, main effect B, and their interaction AB. Of course, ANOVA can be extended to more than two factors, rendering ANOVA a very flexible tool.

Table 9.5 Full presentation of the results of a two-way ANOVA

Source of variance	df	SS	MS	F	p
Effect A (sleep deprivation)	2	125.07	62.53	20.06	<.001
Effect B (age group)	1	40.83	40.83	13.10	<.001
Interaction AB	2	24.27	12.14	3.89	.034
Within (error)	24	74.80	3.12		

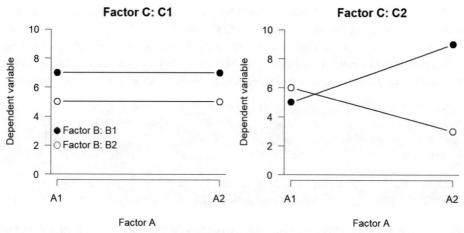

Fig. 9.3 Illustration of a three-way interaction *ABC*. Under the first level of factor *C* (left panel), no interaction *AB* is present, but this is the case under the second level of factor *C* (right panel)

Which pairs of hypotheses can we test in a three-factorial design with the factors *A*, *B*, and *C*? First, there are three main effect hypotheses *A*, *B*, and *C*. Then, each factor can interact with any other factor, so there are three hypotheses about 1st-order interactions (i.e., about two-way interactions): *AB*, *AC*, and *BC*. Finally, and this is new, there is also a 2nd-order interaction: the three-way interaction *ABC*. A significant three-way interaction means that the 1st order interactions differ depending on the level of the third factor. We have illustrated such a case in Fig. 9.3 as an example: While there is *no* interaction of the factors *A* and *B* under the first level of factor *C* (left panel of the figure), these two factors interact under the second level of factor *C* (right panel of the figure).

In sum, we can already test seven pairs of hypotheses in a three-factorial design, and the corresponding decomposition into sums of squares is:

$$SS_{\text{tot}} = SS_A + SS_B + SS_C + SS_{AB} + SS_{AC} + SS_{BC} + SS_{ABC} + SS_w.$$

Practically, however, it is fair to say that ANOVA with three factors can still be interpreted relatively naturally; with more than three factors, interpretation can become challenging.

9.4 Examples and Exercises

9.4.1 Factorial ANOVA with R

We directly use the R package `ez` here to calculate a two-way ANOVA; the calculation with the function `aov()` is described in the online material in the script `9_ANOVA_factorial.R`.

As with the one-way ANOVA (Chap. 8), the data must be available as a data frame (we call it again data) and the data from Table 8.2 is provided in the file 8_data_ANOVA_Sleep deprivation.dat in the online material. From these data, we calculate a new variable age_group from the (existing) variable age, which divides the sample into younger and older adults. We then factorize all relevant variables:

```
# create new variable age_group
data$age_group[data$age < 40] <- 1
data$age_group[data$age >= 40] <- 2
# factorize
data$age_group <- as.factor(data$age_group)
data$sleep_deprivation <- as.factor(data$sleep_deprivation)
data$subject <- as.factor(data$subject)
```

The ANOVA is then calculated again with the function ezANOVA() (see Sect. 8.6.1), but we now specify two (between-subject) factors:

```
ez_result <- ezANOVA(data,
                     wid = .(subject),
                     dv = .(recalled_words),
                     between = .(sleep_deprivation,
                                 age_group),
                     detailed = TRUE)
```

Three- and multi-factorial designs are calculated as well if additional factors are specified. The output ez_result contains all required information to report the tests of the two main effects and the interaction. The total output can again be formatted and reduced with the function anova_out(), which also provides η_p^2 as a measure of effect size:

```
anova_out(ez_result)

$`--- FORMATTED RESULTS --------------------------------`
             Effect                                        Text
1 sleep_deprivation F(2,24) = 20.06, p < .001, np2 = .63
2         age_group F(1,24) = 13.10, p = .001, np2 = .35
3                IA F(2,24) =  3.89, p = .034, np2 = .24
```

Thus, there is a significant main effect of the factor sleep deprivation, $F(2, 24) = 20.06$, $p < .001$, $\eta_p^2 = .63$, as well as of age group, $F(1, 24) = 13.10$, $p = .001$, $\eta_p^2 = .35$. Moreover, the interaction of the two factors is also significant, $F(2, 24) = 3.89$, $p = .034$, $\eta_p^2 = .24$ (the latter shows as sleep_deprivation: age_ group in the original R output; we have abbreviated the interaction to IA in the output to display the results compactly).

To obtain a quick overview of the means of the individual conditions, we can use the functions ezStats() (returning the condition means) and ezPlot() (for a rough graphical representation of the condition means). Both functions follow the same structure as `ezANOVA()`. For `ezPlot()`, additional arguments are required to specify which factor to plot on the x-axis (`x = . (sleep_deprivation)`) and which factor to draw as separate lines for each level (`split = . (age_group)`).

9.4.2 Factorial ANOVA with SPSS

To evaluate the data from Table 8.2 with a two-way ANOVA with SPSS, we open the file `8_data_ANOVA_sleep_deprivation.sav` and prepare the data accordingly. In particular, we calculate a new variable `age_group`, which takes the value 1 if `age` < 40 and the value 2 if `age` ≥ 40. This can be done with the menu

```
Transform > Recode into Different Variables...
```

where we move the original variable (`Age`) into the field *Input Variable→ Output Variable*. In the field *Output Variable* to the right, we enter `Age_Group` as the name of the variable to be created and confirm this with clicking on *Change*. The individual values of the new variable are now determined via the menu *Old and New Values*. For our purposes, we can, for example, use *Range, SMALLEST to Value* and enter 39 as the value. Finally, in the field *New value* a 1 is entered and confirmed with a click on *Add*. Similarly, we can use *Range, Value to HIGHEST* to assign all persons who are at least 40 years old the value 2 on the new variable `Age_Group`.

After this preparatory step, we can now request the ANOVA. For this, we use the menu item

```
Analyze > General Linear Model > Univariate...
```

We are already familiar with the dialog box that appears from the example for the one-way ANOVA (see Fig. 8.8). Here, we move the dependent variable (`Recalled_Words`) into the corresponding field and the two factors (`Sleep_Deprivation` and `Age_Group`) into the field *Fixed Factor(s)*. Additional outputs (descriptive statistics, estimates of effect sizes, plots) can be requested as described for the one-way ANOVA (see Sect. 8.6.2). The inferential statistical results can then be found in the table *Tests of Between-Subjects Effects* (Fig. 9.4). In our case, there is a significant main effect of the factor sleep deprivation, $F(2, 24) = 20.06$, $p < .001$, $\eta_p^2 = .63$, as well as of age group, $F(1, 24) = 13.10$, $p = .001$, $\eta_p^2 = .35$. Moreover, the interaction of the two factors is significant, $F(2, 24) = 3.89$, $p = .034$, $\eta_p^2 = .24$. The degrees of freedom can be obtained from separate rows, using the row for which the first column indicates the effect of interest and the row indicated by *Error*.

Tests of Between-Subjects Effects

Dependent Variable: Recalled_Words

Source	Type III Sum of Squares	df	Mean Square	F	Sig.	Partial Eta Squared
Corrected Model	190.167[a]	5	38.033	12.203	.000	.718
Intercept	7332.033	1	7332.033	2352.524	.000	.990
Sleep_Deprivation	125.067	2	62.533	20.064	.000	.626
Age_Group	40.833	1	40.833	13.102	.001	.353
Sleep_Deprivation * Age_Group	24.267	2	12.133	3.893	.034	.245
Error	74.800	24	3.117			
Total	7597.000	30				
Corrected Total	264.967	29				

a. R Squared = .718 (Adjusted R Squared = .659)

Fig. 9.4 Output of a two-way ANOVA with SPSS

Repeated-Measures Analysis of Variance (ANOVA) 10

In the introductory example for the one-way analysis of variance (ANOVA; see Chap. 8), we had different groups treated with one of the three levels of the factor "duration of sleep deprivation". We used this example to motivate the view of one-way ANOVA as generalizing the independent-samples t-test to more than two samples.

From Chap. 5 we also know the t-test for two *dependent* samples already. This test is applied when each person provides values for both conditions. Now, we could also conduct an investigation of the effect of sleep deprivation on memory performance in such a way that each tested person completes a memory test without sleep deprivation *and* after 1 day, and after 2 days of sleep deprivation. Each person then provides three data points, and to analyze such data we need the **repeated-measures ANOVA**—in a sense, the generalization of the t-test for two dependent samples (or conditions) to more than two dependent samples (or conditions). The focus is then again on the condition-dependent changes within each tested person; this is why it also is called a within-subject ANOVA.

To understand the principle of repeated-measures ANOVA, we first consider a simplified method of its calculation. We then turn to the general procedure for repeated-measures ANOVA with a single factor, which is very similar to the two-way ANOVA as introduced in Chap. 9.

10.1 A Simple Approach to Repeated-Measures ANOVA

We now consider the data of the younger adults from Table 9.1 and imagine that the values of each row come from one person each (see the left part of Table 10.1).[1]

---

[1] A close look shows that we did not use the exact same data here. In fact, the values of each column are the same, but we scrambled their order slightly. This was done to avoid the impression that one

© Springer-Verlag GmbH Germany, part of Springer Nature 2023
M. Janczyk, R. Pfister, *Understanding Inferential Statistics*,
https://doi.org/10.1007/978-3-662-66786-6_10

Table 10.1 Example data for a repeated-measures ANOVA with one single factor.

	Sleep deprivation					Sleep deprivation			
Person	0 days	1 day	2 days	M	Person	0 days	1 day	2 days	M
1	22	18	17	19.0	1	3	-1	-2	0.0
2	18	17	16	17.0	2	1	0	-1	0.0
3	19	17	16	17.3	3	1.67	-0.33	-1.33	0.0
4	18	16	15	16.3	4	1.67	-0.33	-1.33	0.0
5	14	16	13	14.3	5	-0.33	1.67	-1.33	0.0
M_j	18.2	16.8	15.4		M_j	1.40	0.00	-1.40	
s_j^2	6.56	0.56	1.84		s_j^2	1.17	0.80	0.11	

From the means of the individual persons we see that they generally differ in their memory performance. However, we are not interested in these inter-individual differences; instead, we are interested in the effect of the factor "sleep deprivation" on memory performance *within* each person. In the example, the overall pattern looks quite similar across individuals (except for person 5).

In order to get rid of the inter-individual differences, we subtract the mean of each person from each measured score of this person (see the right part of Table 10.1). These new scores are called **ipsative scores** and their major property is that the mean of each subject is now 0. In other words, the subjects do not differ in their general level of performance any longer, because the existing inter-individual differences—in which we are not interested at this stage—have been eliminated. However, the pattern of differences between the three levels *within* each person remains the same.

For further illustration, we now calculate a one-way ANOVA for the original and for the ipsative scores.[2] For the original scores, the slight decrease in performance with increasing sleep deprivation is not significant, $F(2, 12) = 2.63$, $p = .113$, but we get a significant result for the ipsative scores, $F(2, 12) = 11.31$, $p = .002$. What is the reason for these different outcomes? The first thing to note is that in both cases we get $SS_A = 19.60$. Thus, the variability due to the (experimental) factor is identical. However, while the error sum of square is $SS_w = 44.80$ for the original data, it is only $SS_w = 10.40$ for the ipsative scores. Since the resulting error term MS_w is in the denominator of the F-ratio, the F-value is larger. Accordingly, eliminating the inter-individual differences increased the power of the test by reducing the error term. In fact, inter-individual differences are a major share of the error term in (standard) ANOVA (see Chap. 8).

---

and the same data set should be treated at will in either the between-subject way or in the within-subject way, while still using familiar data that yield the same condition means and variances.

[2] The detailed calculations are presented in the online material.

In Depth 10.1: A Note on Evaluating Ipsative Score

In the introductory example we have pretended that we can compute a "normal" one-way ANOVA on the ipsative scores. Against this background it appears tempting to use the F-distribution with $(J - 1)$ and $(N - J)$ degrees of freedom to evaluate the findings, where N is the number of data points. However, the (ipsative) scores are not independent of each other, whereas independence is a main assumption of the (normal) one-way ANOVA. Strictly speaking, therefore, the denominator degrees of freedom must be reduced to $(J - 1)(N - 1)$, where N is the number of persons tested. Although this increases the critical F-value, the simultaneous increase in the empirical F-value due to eliminating the inter-individual differences outweighs this effect in most cases.

10.2 Dealing with Inter-Individual Differences

To illustrate the rationale of a repeated-measures ANOVA, we "eliminated" inter-individual differences by using ipsative scores in the previous section. The actual repeated-measures ANOVA employs a very similar procedure that is more flexible, however: The inter-individual differences are considered a separate effect that is quantified in the same way as the actual effects of interest. By this, the associated variability is attributed to a factor, even though the effect of the inter-individual differences is rarely of interest and is ultimately ignored. Thus, a repeated-measures ANOVA with one factor is very similar to a standard two-way ANOVA (Chap. 9). The first factor A is the effect of interest with J levels, and the second factor is called subject (S) and it has as many levels as there are participants in the sample (i.e., N). It follows that each design cell comprises exactly one value in this case.

The formulas required are those we introduced in Sect. 9.2 already: We determine SS_A, SS_S, as well as SS_{AS}, and use them to compute the corresponding mean sums of squares by dividing them by the respective degrees of freedom. Let us now ignore the inter-individual differences SS_S and consider the remaining sums of squares, except for SS_A, as contributing to the error term, that is $SS_{error} = SS_{AS} + SS_w$. A noteworthy observation arises from the fact that each design cell comprises only one data point, so that there is no variance within each cell and thus $SS_w = 0$. Therefore, we are eventually left with $SS_{error} = SS_{AS}$. The interaction of factor A and the subject factor S is thus the basis for the error term in the F-ratio of the repeated-measures ANOVA:

$$F = \frac{MS_A}{MS_{AS}}.$$

One can also show that, if the H_0 is assumed to be true (i.e., identical population means in all conditions), this F-ratio is F-distributed with $J - 1$ numerator degrees of freedom and

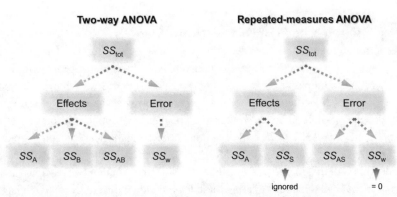

Fig. 10.1 Decomposition of the sums of squares for a two-way ANOVA (left panel) and a repeated-measures ANOVA with one single factor (right panel). SS_S quantifies the part of the total variability that is due to inter-individual differences and is eventually ignored; SS_w is always 0 in a repeated-measures ANOVA, because each design cell comprises only one value. Thus, the interaction between factor A and the subject factor S remains as the error term

$(J - 1)(N - 1)$ denominator degrees of freedom. The decision rule and the interpretation of the decision then correspond to all forms of ANOVA discussed in the previous chapters.

To illustrate the similarities, we have compared the decomposition of the sums of squares for the two-way ANOVA and the repeated-measures ANOVA with one single factor in Fig. 10.1.

10.3 Dependent vs. Independent Samples

Some research questions can only be studied with independent samples in a meaningful way, for example, comparing men and women with respect to a particular variable. There are also research questions that can only be addressed meaningfully with dependent samples. An example of this would be the well-being of people before and after a therapy or other intervention. Accordingly, there are cases where the use of independent or dependent samples is already determined by the question at hand. If there is a choice between the two options though, several aspects are worth considering, such as the *availability of participants* and the *duration* of a single condition: If participants are easily available and each condition takes a long time to complete, a design with independent samples may sometimes be preferable. However, if there are few suitable participants, and each condition takes little time on its own, this situation calls for designs with dependent samples.

The most important advantage of dependent samples, as evaluated, for example, with a repeated-measures ANOVA, is the increase in the empirical F-value as a direct consequence of reducing the error term. In other words, the power of the test increases when working with dependent samples. Especially in experimental (cognitive) psychology, the differences between persons are usually quite large, whereas the effects of interest are rather subtle. Corresponding studies therefore lean towards using dependent samples.

An important aspect of dependent samples are potential **sequence effects**. These effects can become problematic if there is a confound of (experimental) conditions (i.e., factor levels) and their temporal order, that is, if the conditions are performed in the same order for all participants. Observing performance to improve in these designs may simply result from practice. Similarly, deterioration may result from fatigue. Related to this are problems that arise when one condition has an effect on the subsequent condition. These may be familiarity with the stimulus material, perceptual adaptation, or much more subtle mechanisms. One measure against such effects is a sufficient time interval between applying the conditions. For more details on appropriate methods for dealing with these problems (e.g., counterbalancing), we refer the reader to Bortz and Schuster (2010) or to Shadish et al. (2002).

10.4 Concluding Remarks

10.4.1 Violations of Assumptions

In case of the ANOVA as described in Chaps. 8 and 9, we assumed independence of the samples. This independence is, of course, violated in case of dependent samples: a faster person will be faster across conditions than a slower person. The different conditions are thus not independent of each other. To still derive the distribution of a corresponding random variable, the following assumption is made instead: The variances of all pairwise differences between the conditions are equal. If this condition is satisfied, this is called **sphericity**.[3] It follows that in the case of a factor with only two levels, sphericity always holds. However, if sphericity is violated in a data set, the repeated-measures ANOVA behaves liberally, that is, there is an increased chance of incorrectly deciding in favor of the H_1.

A common test of the sphericity assumption is Mauchly's W-test (Mauchly 1940), which often appears in the output of computer programs. The important point here is: If the test is significant, this is evidence *against* the assumption of sphericity. In this case, we can estimate the magnitude of the violation, and this estimate is denoted by ϵ (a lowercase epsilon) and it can take values between 0 and 1. This estimate can be used to adjust the degrees of freedom of the respective F-ratio by multiplying the original degrees of freedom with ϵ. The degrees of freedom thus become smaller and the resulting critical F-value increases, counteracting the liberality. There are various methods for estimating ϵ. One commonly recommended way was introduced by Greenhouse and Geisser (1959) and is

---

[3] If the data comply with **compound symmetry**, that is, all variances are equal and all pairwise covariances (see Chap. 11) are equal, sphericity is implied by this (for more information, see Maxwell et al. 2018, and Lane 2016).

often part of the output of computer programs. Non-parametric alternatives to the ANOVA with repeated measures are the Friedman rank ANOVA or the Kendall W test (see, e.g., Bortz and Schuster 2010; Howell 2017).

10.4.2 Effect Sizes

The same effect sizes are generally used for repeated-measures ANOVA as were introduced in the two previous chapters. The only thing to note when estimating them is to use the correct error term, that is, the interaction of the subject factor with the factor of interest.

10.4.3 Confidence Intervals

Adequate procedures for calculating confidence intervals with dependent samples have been discussed quite intensely in recent years (Baguley 2012; Bakeman and McArthur 1996; Cousineau 2017; Franz and Loftus 2012; Loftus and Masson 1994; Pfister and Janczyk 2013). The most influential proposal for calculating confidence intervals in case of (more than two) dependent samples goes back to Loftus and Masson (1994). According to this approach, the corresponding confidence interval is calculated analogously to the one used in standard ANOVA (see Sect. 8.5.2) and is therefore based on the error term MS_{AS}:

$$\left[M_j \pm t_{(J-1)(N-1); \frac{\alpha}{2}} \cdot \sqrt{\frac{MS_{AS}}{n}} \right].$$

Then, two means M_k and M_m differ significantly from each other if

$$|M_k - M_m| > \sqrt{2} \cdot t_{(J-1)(N-1); \frac{\alpha}{2}} \cdot \sqrt{\frac{MS_{AS}}{n}} \qquad k, m \in \{1, \dots, J\}.$$

10.4.4 Multi-Factor Repeated-Measures ANOVA

Of course, we can also perform multi-factor repeated-measures ANOVA. This combines the advantages of multi-factor designs (e.g., studying interactions) and dependent samples (e.g., higher power). To do this, consider the example of a repeated-measures ANOVA with the two factors A and B. Similar to a standard ANOVA, we can then test three hypotheses: main effects A and B, and their interaction AB.

Remember that we treated the repeated-measures ANOVA with one factor as a standard two-way ANOVA (see Sect. 10.2) and introduced the subject factor S as the second factor. We now treat the repeated-measures ANOVA with two factors as a standard three-way ANOVA (see Sect. 9.3.4). The three factors are therefore A, B, and the subject factor S. The only difference to the standard two-way ANOVA is the type of error terms used: Whereas in the standard ANOVA, we always used MS_w in the denominator of the F-ratios, in the repeated measures case, we always use the interaction of the subject factor with the relevant factor. We therefore use different error terms for each of the three F-ratios and, accordingly, usually use different F-distributions in each case for the decisions as well:

$$F^A = \frac{MS_A}{MS_{AS}}, \qquad F^B = \frac{MS_B}{MS_{BS}} \quad \text{and} \quad F^{AB} = \frac{MS_{AB}}{MS_{ABS}}.$$

10.4.5 Mixed ANOVA

Consider again the introductory example and imagine that we had included older adults as well and exposed each of them to the three conditions of sleep deprivation. While sleep deprivation would still be a factor with repeated measures, age group, in contrast, is a factor without repeated measures, of course. The case of (at least) one factor realized with dependent samples and (at least) one other factor realized with independent samples requires so-called **mixed ANOVA**. The general procedure is identical to other ANOVAs described in this book. Further details can be found, for example, in Keppel and Wickens (2004).

10.5 Examples and Exercises

10.5.1 Repeated-Measures ANOVA with R

To run a repeated-measures ANOVA, we here use the package ez. The calculation with the function aov() is described in the online material in the script 10_ANOVA_repeated_measures.R. In the following, we assume that the data from Table 10.1 (10_data_ANOVA_repeated_measures.dat) were read and assigned to a data frame named data. After factorizing the relevant variables, we pass this data frame to the ezANOVA() function. The only difference is that the variable `sleep_deprivation` is now labeled as a variable with repeated measures by using `within = .(...)`:[4]

```
data$subject <- as.factor(data$subject)
data$sleep_deprivation <- as.factor(data$sleep_deprivation)
ez_result <- ezANOVA(data,
                     wid = .(subject),
                     dv = .(recalled_words),
                     within = .(sleep_deprivation),
                     detailed = TRUE)
ez_result
```

The results are provided in three tables:

```
$ANOVA
             Effect DFn DFd    SSn  SSd           F ...
1        (Intercept)   1   4 4233.6 34.4 492.279070 ...
2 sleep_deprivation   2   8   19.6 10.4   7.538462 ...
                               ...p p<0.05        ges
                      ...2.442699e-05     *  0.9895288
                      ...1.444270e-02     *  0.3043478


$'Mauchly's Test for Sphericity'
             Effect         W            p p<0.05
2 sleep_deprivation 0.1873767 0.08110983


$'Sphericity Corrections'
             Effect       GGe       p[GG] p[GG]<0.05 ...
2 sleep_deptivation 0.5516866 0.04507414          * ...
                          ...HFe       p[HF] p[HF]<0.05
                     ...0.6070624 0.03903435          *
```

The first table `$ANOVA` summarizes the results of the ANOVA under the assumption of sphericity. By default, `ez` provides generalized η^2 as the effect size (column *ges*), which leads to values different than η_p^2 (see also Footnote 8 in Chap. 8). The online material describes how to calculate η_p^2 from the output of `ez`. For the example data, there is a significant effect of the factor sleep deprivation, $F(2, 8) = 7.54$, $p = .014$, $\eta_p^2 = .65$. Then, in the second table, we find Mauchly's test for sphericity. It is not significant here, $p = .081$, which means we continue to assume sphericity. If this were not true, we could use the values of the third table that provides corrected results; GG refers to the

---

[4] Unlike for SPSS (see Sect. 10.5.2), it is not necessary to arrange variables with repeated measures in different columns per level.

Greenhouse-Geisser correction and HF to an alternative correction by Huynh-Feldt. Again, the output can be formatted and condensed with

```
anova_out(ez_result)
```

which also gives an estimate of η_p^2. In addition, anova_out() provides information about tests of the sphericity assumption and corrects p-values automatically if required.

In addition, if a factor without repeated measures is present in our design (see Sect. 10.4.5), ezANOVA() can easily be called with the additional argument between = .(...) to specify the corresponding mixed ANOVA. This may yield different results than the SPSS calculation in case of unequal sample sizes, because different types of sums of squares are calculated (see Box 9.2). In order to obtain the same results, we need to use the argument type = 3.

10.5.2 Repeated-Measures ANOVA with SPSS

The file 10_data_ANOVA_repeated_measures.sav provides the data from Table 10.1 and comprises three lines for each person. In each of these rows, we find the number of recalled words in one of the three conditions corresponding to 0, 1, or 2 days of sleep deprivation. SPSS requires the levels of a factor with repeated measures as separate variables (i.e., as separate columns). We thus need to prepare the data for further analysis, and convert the (condition) rows into columns via the menu

```
Data > Restructure...
```

We select the middle option *Restructuring selected cases into variables* and move the variable Subject into the field *Identifier Variable(s)*, and the variable Sleep_Deprivation into the field *Index Variable(s)*. Then we click *Next* and select the *Use data as currently sorted* option. After confirming with *Finish*, we see that each person's data are now listed in a single row. The repeated-measures ANOVA can now be selected via the menu

```
Analyze > General Linear Model > Repeated Measures...
```

In the dialog box, we label the (single) factor Sleep_Deprivation and specify that it has three levels. Clicking on *Define* then brings us to the next dialog box (Fig. 10.2, left panel). There, we move the three variables, which now represent the three levels of the factor (Recalled_Words.0 etc.), into the three placeholders of the field *Within-Subjects Variables*.

With the dialog box behind the field *Options*, we can again request, for example, descriptive statistics and estimators for effect sizes (η_p^2) to be provided in the output (Fig. 10.2, right panel). Similar to the previous chapters, the graphical output can be

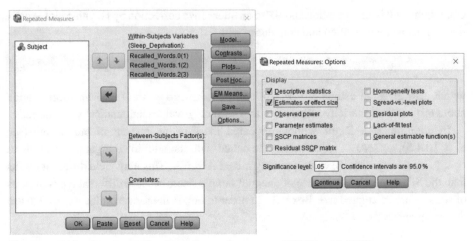

Fig. 10.2 Dialog box for performing a repeated-measures ANOVA with SPSS

Mauchly's Test of Sphericity[a]

Measure: MEASURE_1

Within Subjects Effect	Mauchly's W	Approx. Chi-Square	df	Sig.	Epsilon[b]		
					Greenhouse-Geisser	Huynh-Feldt	Lower-bound
Sleep_Deprivation	.187	5.024	2	.081	.552	.607	.500

Tests the null hypothesis that the error covariance matrix of the orthonormalized transformed dependent variables is proportional to an identity matrix.

   a. Design: Intercept
      Within Subjects Design: Sleep_Deprivation

   b. May be used to adjust the degrees of freedom for the averaged tests of significance. Corrected tests are
      displayed in the Tests of Within-Subjects Effects table.

Tests of Within-Subjects Effects

Measure: MEASURE_1

Source		Type III Sum of Squares	df	Mean Square	F	Sig.	Partial Eta Squared
Sleep_Deprivation	Sphericity Assumed	19.600	2	9.800	7.538	.014	.653
	Greenhouse-Geisser	19.600	1.103	17.764	7.538	.045	.653
	Huynh-Feldt	19.600	1.214	16.143	7.538	.039	.653
	Lower-bound	19.600	1.000	19.600	7.538	.052	.653
Error(Sleep_Deprivation)	Sphericity Assumed	10.400	8	1.300			
	Greenhouse-Geisser	10.400	4.413	2.356			
	Huynh-Feldt	10.400	4.856	2.141			
	Lower-bound	10.400	4.000	2.600			

Fig. 10.3 Output of a repeated-measures ANOVA with SPSS

specified in the menu *Plots*. The actual output (Fig. 10.3) comprises a larger number of tables. The most important information for us, the inferential statistical results, are provided in the table *Tests of Within-Subjects Effects*: For all factors with repeated measures and for the interactions involving these factors, we find all relevant statistics such as F, p, and η_p^2 (we will focus on the values in the row labeled *Sphericity Assumed* for now). The degrees of freedom for the F-ratio can be taken from the respective rows of the factor of interest and the row *Error*. For our example, we obtain a significant effect of the factor sleep deprivation, $F(2, 8) = 7.54$, $p = .014$, $\eta_p^2 = .65$.

Another important part of the output is shown in the table labeled *Mauchly Test of Sphericity*. These are the tests about whether sphericity can be assumed or whether appropriate corrections should be used. With $p = .081$, we stick with the sphericity assumption. The three columns labeled *Epsilon* estimate the extent of a violation of sphericity in different ways. If Mauchly's test was significant, the p-value of the ANOVA would have to be corrected accordingly. Corrections, such as the one suggested by Greenhouse-Geisser, can be found in the table *Tests of Within-Subjects Effects*. In case there is also a factor without repeated measures in our design (see Sect. 10.4.5), we can use the field *Between-Subjects Factors* to specify a mixed ANOVA.

Correlation and Regression

11

The test procedures introduced across the preceding chapters aimed at testing difference hypotheses. This type of hypotheses already covers a wide range of scientific questions and research designs. It does not cover the relevant topic of **correlation hypotheses**, however (see Sect. 4.1.1).

To get a sense of this approach, we first need to clarify what a statistical relationship (or statistical dependence) actually is. In particular, the statistical notion of (in)dependence of two or more variables is a separate concept that can be easily confused with the (unrelated) concept of independent and dependent variables in the context of experimental design. Building on the concept of statistical (in)dependence, we will derive a measure to describe linear relationships in the second section. The third section then introduces simple linear regression, which is another way of assessing the relationship between two variables. In the last section, we give a short outlook on more advanced concepts such as multiple regression and partial correlation.

11.1 Relationship and Dependence of Variables

Scientific reports often claim that two "variables are related" or that one variable is "dependent on another variable". Corresponding correlation hypotheses form the second group of statistical hypotheses in addition to the difference hypotheses that we have looked at so far. However, the concept of dependence in statistics does not map entirely on the colloquial use of the word.

What do statistical dependence and independence mean? To illustrate, let us imagine that two variables were collected from 60 persons: their gender and the number of tattoos (1 vs. 2 vs. 3). The left part of Table 11.1 shows the absolute frequencies of each combination. In this example, each combination occurred with equal frequency, that is,

© Springer-Verlag GmbH Germany, part of Springer Nature 2023
M. Janczyk, R. Pfister, *Understanding Inferential Statistics*,
https://doi.org/10.1007/978-3-662-66786-6_11

Table 11.1 Example results of a study that recorded the two variables "gender" and "number of tattoos" for a sample of $n = 60$ tattooed persons. Individual cells show absolute frequencies

Gender	Tattoos				Gender	Tattoos			
	1	2	3	$\sum$		1	2	3	$\sum$
Male	10	10	10	30	Male	15	0	15	30
Female	10	10	10	30	Female	0	30	0	30
$\sum$	20	20	20	60	$\sum$	15	30	15	60

knowing the gender of a single person does not help to specify the number of their tattoos. This is also true in the reverse direction, that is, if we want to infer a person's gender from the number of tattoos. This is an example of what we call **complete independence**.

But what if we had obtained a result as shown in the right part of Table 11.1? In this case, we can perfectly determine the gender of a person from knowing the number of tattoos. We call this case **complete dependence.** A notable peculiarity of the statistical meaning of dependence is that perfect determination only has to work in one direction for us to speak of complete dependence. Thus, it is sufficient to be able to determine gender perfectly from the number of tattoos, but it is not necessary to be able to specify the number of tattoos equally perfectly from gender.

Statistical dependencies (or "relations" to use a common synonym) have two important properties; their type and their strength:

- **Type of relation:** A relation between two variables can come in many different forms. Examples include linear relationships and U-shaped quadratic relationships (see Fig. 11.1). Of course, many other types of relations are conceivable just as well.
- **Strength of the relation:** Complete dependence and complete independence are two poles of a continuum with infinitely many levels in between. In the following section, we will learn about one measure that describes the strength of a linear relationship.

11.2   The (Bivariate) Correlation Coefficient

Our goal in this section is to find a measure that reaches a certain maximum with complete linear dependence and a certain minimum with complete linear independence of two variables. The so-called bivariate correlation, Pearson product-moment correlation, or simply correlation coefficient is suitable for this purpose. We will illustrate its derivation with a graphical approach first and then discuss how to compute a statistical test for the correlation coefficient.

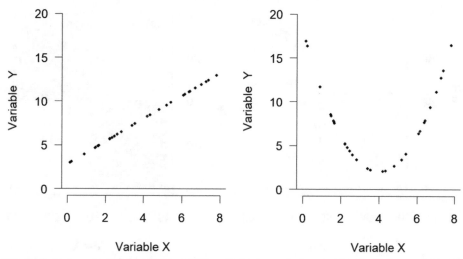

Fig. 11.1 Types of relations of two variables. The left panel shows a linear relation and the right panel shows a U-shaped, quadratic relation

11.2.1 Derivation and Calculation

For the following considerations, let us assume that we have tested $n = 100$ persons, each on two tests designed to measure the same ability. A maximum score of 80 can be obtained in each test. The left panel of Fig. 11.2 shows the resulting data as a scatterplot, with each point corresponding to one particular person. The figure also shows the *centroid* of the data as a large black dot. This is the point with the coordinates M_X and M_Y, that is, the means of the x- and y-coordinates of all data points. It can be seen in the figure that high x-scores (Test A) tend to be accompanied by high y-scores (Test B), but the points do not lie on a straight line either. For now, let us agree that this is a "linear and positive" relationship, albeit not a perfect one.

To understand the construction of the correlation coefficient, it is helpful to move the origin of the coordinate system to the centroid. We have done this in the right part of Fig. 11.2, which also highlights the four quadrants of the coordinate system (Q1–Q4). In this coordinate system, the coordinates x and y of the data points indicate the deviations of the measured score from the means M_X and M_Y of both variables.

Now we first consider those data points located in the 1st and 3rd quadrant. For these data, the deviations of the x-coordinate from M_X and the y-coordinate from M_Y always have the same sign: In quadrant 1, they are both positive, and in quadrant 3, they are both

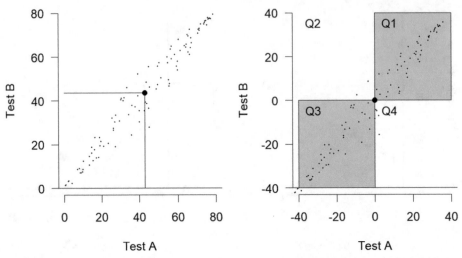

Fig. 11.2 Data of $n = 100$ persons in a coordinate system including the centroid of the data. The left panel shows the raw data and the right panel shows shifted values to align the origin of the coordinate system with the centroid

negative. Hence, the product of both deviations is always positive:

$$(x_i - M_X) \cdot (y_i - M_Y) > 0 \quad \forall i \in \{1, \ldots, n\} \qquad \text{in quadrants 1 and 3.}$$

For all data points in the 2nd and 4th quadrant, on the other hand, one deviation is always positive, the other negative. The product of both deviations is thus always negative:

$$(x_i - M_X) \cdot (y_i - M_Y) < 0 \quad \forall i \in \{1, \ldots, n\} \qquad \text{in quadrants 2 and 4.}$$

Based on this pattern, we consider the sum of these products across all the n persons and call this sum G:

$$G = \sum_{i=1}^{n} (x_i - M_X) \cdot (y_i - M_Y). \tag{11.1}$$

From the above considerations, it follows that points in quadrants 1 and 3 contribute positive scores, whereas points in quadrants 2 and 4 contribute negative scores to G. Thus, if more (and more extreme) data points lie in quadrants 1 and 3, then G becomes positive; but if there are more (and more extreme) data points in quadrants 2 and 4, then G becomes negative.

We have noted above that the pattern in Fig. 11.2 indicates a positive correlation. Thus, most points lie in quadrants 1 and 3, and this is also where the more extreme points lie, that is, those with large deviations from the centroid. As a consequence, the total sum G becomes positive. With similar considerations, we see that G would become negative, if the scatterplot was to show data points stretching from quadrant 2 to quadrant 4. Finally, G would approach 0, if the data points were equally distributed among all four quadrants, so that the scatterplot would have a circular shape, for example.

The sum G of products of deviations (Eq. 11.1) appears to be a reasonable measure for the strength of the (linear) relation of two variables: It becomes more *positive*, the more larger values on one variable are accompanied by larger values on the other variable. At the same time, it becomes more *negative*, the more larger values on one variable are associated with smaller values on the other variable. Finally, a value around 0 results when the data points are equally distributed across the four quadrants. To enable a comparison of G across different sample sizes, we further divide G by n. The resulting measure is called the **covariance** of the two variables X and Y:

$$\text{Cov}(X, Y) = \frac{1}{n} \sum_{i=1}^{n} (x_i - M_X)(y_i - M_Y).$$

Some *important properties of the covariance* are:

- $\text{Cov}(X, Y) = \text{Cov}(Y, X)$
- The covariance of a variable with itself is its variance: $\text{Cov}(X, X) = S_X^2$.
- For statistically independent variables, the covariance is zero. In other words: If X and Y are statistically independent, then $\text{Cov}(X, Y) = 0$. Importantly, the reverse conclusion does *not* hold! From $\text{Cov}(X, Y) = 0$, we cannot conclude that both variables are fully independent of each other; they are only *linearly* independent, but may exhibit other types of dependencies.
- Two measured variables are typically neither completely independent of one another, nor are they completely dependent. Hence, it is important to know what minimum and maximum the covariance can theoretically take in case of complete dependence. It is possible to show that in case of a complete, linear, and negative dependence, the covariance reaches a minimum of $-S_X S_Y$; for a complete, linear, and positive dependence, it reaches a maximum of $+S_X S_Y$ (S_X and S_Y are the standard deviations of X and Y; for more details, see the online material). Thus, the value range of the covariance of two variables X and Y is:

$$-S_X S_Y \leq \text{Cov}(X, Y) \leq S_X S_Y. \tag{11.2}$$

When we additionally perform a standardization[1] by dividing this inequality by $S_X S_Y$, we ensure that this new measure can only vary between -1 and 1:

$$-1 \leq \frac{\text{Cov}(X, Y)}{S_X S_Y} \leq 1.$$

This measure is called the **correlation coefficient** r:

$$r_{XY} = \frac{\text{Cov}(X, Y)}{S_X S_Y}. \tag{11.3}$$

With r_{XY} we thus have a measure reflecting the strength of a linear relationship between two variables that does not depend on the unit of measurement of the data.[2] We can therefore indicate the strength of a linear relationship in a given sample. While $r = 0$ indicates no linear relationship, $r = -1$ and $r = 1$ correspond to a perfect linear relationship. In case of $r = -1$, this relationship is negative, and in case of $r = 1$, it is positive. We now turn to the question of what we can conclude from this coefficient about the correlation in the population.

In Depth 11.1: The Correlation Coefficient as an Effect Size

For difference hypotheses we had computed separate measures of effect size that standardized observed differences relative to a suitable measure of variability. This extra step is not necessary for correlations, because r already is an estimator of the effect size of the correlation in the population. There are also conventions proposed by Cohen (1988) to label the strength of a correlation based on categories. Here, $|r| = 0.10$, $|r| = 0.30$, and $|r| = 0.50$ are the lower bounds to consider an effect as small, medium, and large, respectively. Meta-analyses also take advantage of the fact that many other effect sizes can be converted (at least approximately) into r.

Another property of r is that r^2 (often denoted as R^2) indicates the proportion of shared variance of both variables and thus comes with a graspable interpretation.

---

[1] In the context of the effect size δ (Sect. 7.2), we had already pointed out that, for example, differences and deviations often change depending on the underlying unit of measurement. To calculate δ, we had therefore divided the difference by the standard deviation σ. Since the property of dependence on the unit of measurement also applies to the covariance, a similar standardization is done here.

[2] So far, we have assumed that the two variables are measured at the level of interval scales. An alternative for ordinal data is, for example, Spearman's ρ (a lowercase rho; Spearman 1910; see also, e.g., Zar 2005). This ρ should not be confused with the population parameter ρ that will be considered soon. Even though both statistics use the same symbol, they refer to distinct concepts.

11.2.2 Inferential Statistics of the Correlation

In general, the correlation coefficient calculated with Formula 11.3 will nearly always be different from 0 in a sample. However, as we have discussed in the context of difference hypotheses, we are usually not interested in the correlation of the two variables in a particular sample, but instead we are interested in the correlation in the underlying population. We denote this population parameter by ρ (a lowercase rho). As with all population parameters considered so far, even if $\rho = 0$, the sample statistic is usually $r \neq 0$. Using an inferential statistical test, we now want to assess whether $r \neq 0$ also indicates that a corresponding correlation exists in the population, that is, if $\rho \neq 0$ as well.

The general procedure follows the same logic as for all the tests discussed so far. We begin with formulating a pair of hypotheses, where the H_0 is again formulated exactly (here for the two-sided case):

$$H_0 : \rho = 0 \quad \text{and} \quad H_1 : \rho \neq 0.$$

Next, we develop a test statistic with the two properties: (1) It should come with more extreme values the more the data speak against the H_0, and (2) the probability density function (or distribution) of a corresponding random variable (which assigns this quantity to every possible sample from the population) should be known if the H_0 were true.

The first point is already true for the correlation coefficient r, whereas this is not the case for the second point. However, both properties are fulfilled by a certain ratio t that is calculated from r and the sample size n:

$$t = \frac{r\sqrt{n-2}}{\sqrt{1-r^2}} \overset{H_0}{\sim} t_{n-2}. \tag{11.4}$$

The remaining steps are just as in the previous tests. We determine the critical t-value, and if our empirical t-value (from Formula 11.4) exceeds the critical value, we know: If the $H_0 : \rho = 0$ was true, the observed data (or more extreme outcomes) are so unlikely that we doubt this assumption and instead decide for the H_1. Formally, the decision rule (here for the two-sided case) is:

Reject the H_0, if $|t| \geq t_{n-2;\frac{\alpha}{2}}$ or if $p \leq \alpha$.

11.3 Simple Linear Regression

In the previous section, we derived the correlation coefficient as a measure for the strength of linear relationships. This measure treated both variables X and Y equally. A related approach is called regression, but in a sense it distinguishes between dependent and independent variables as is commonly done in experimental design. In this section, we will discuss **simple linear regression**, which only includes one independent variable.

As a visual metaphor, simple linear regression is about drawing a straight line through the points of a scatterplot that best represents the data. Of course, we will need to clarify what "best" means in this context. But why do need regression at all?

- Empirical data often cannot be collected until the observations cover the whole range of a variable. However, by means of such a regression line, we could make informed guesses about which y-value a person with a particular x-value would have. In other words, we can *predict* the values on one variable from the value on the other variable. For this reason, the (independent) variable used for prediction in the context of regression is also called the **predictor**, and the predicted (dependent) variable is called the **criterion**.
- Relationships sometimes follow mathematical functions—and they do so more or less exactly. Often, but by far not always, these relationships are linear, that is, they can be described by a straight line. If we consider the deviations of the empirical values from this theoretical straight line the result of *measurement error*, we would have an idea of the "true" relationship (i.e., without measurement error).

11.3.1 Determining a Regression Line

How do we determine the equation of that particular straight line that "best represents" the data? Suppose we had a sample of $n = 6$ persons who provided data on two variables X and Y, that is, $(x_1, y_1), \ldots, (x_6, y_6)$. Figure 11.3 shows these data as a scatterplot along with a straight line passing through the data. A straight line is mathematically described by a function of the form $f(x) = bx + a$, where b is the slope of the line and a its intercept, that is, the point of intersection with the y-axis. The goal of the following section is finding suitable values for b and a.

Let us assume that we already know the straight line we are looking for. Then, for each data point x_i, we could use the function to calculate a predicted value $f(x_i)$ that, of course, lies on the straight line. If we denote these *predicted* y-values with $\hat{y}$, they can be described as:

$$\hat{y}_i = bx_i + a \qquad \forall i \in \{1, \ldots, n\}.$$

Deviations of the predicted values from the measured values, that is,

$$e_i = y_i - \hat{y}_i \, ,$$

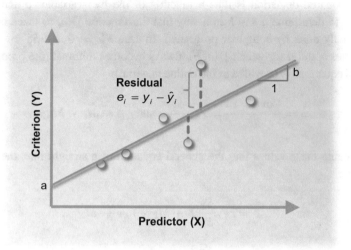

Fig. 11.3 Scatterplot of $n = 6$ data points with a regression line as described by the function $f(x) = bx + a$. The vertical difference of a data point y_i from the value predicted by the straight line, $\hat{y}_i$, is called the residual e_i

are referred to as **residuals** e_i (see Fig. 11.3). To best describe the actual y_i via the (predicted) $\hat{y}_i$ values, we should choose the straight line in such a way, that the residuals e_i become as small as possible.

The next question is: What is an appropriate overall measure of deviation of observed and predicted values? If we simply calculate all residuals e_i and sum them up, they cancel each other out. Therefore, we instead consider the sum of the absolute deviations or, even better, the sum of the squared deviations. Usually, the total deviation measure used is the *squared deviation Q*:

$$Q = \sum_{i=1}^{n} e_i^2 = \sum_{i=1}^{n} (y_i - \hat{y}_i)^2 \tag{11.5}$$

A straight line thus represents the data "as best as possible" if Q becomes as small as possible without any other straight line producing even smaller values for Q. This is called the method of **(ordinary) least squares** (sometimes abbreviated as OLS). To determine the parameters b and a, we substitute for $\hat{y}_i$ the general function of a straight line and rewrite Formula 11.5 as:

$$Q(a, b) = \sum_{i=1}^{n} (y_i - (bx_i + a))^2.$$

The mean squared deviation is thus a function of the two variables a and b, and the objective is to determine a and b in a way that the function $Q(a, b)$ takes its minimum (this is usually done by computer programs). In case $S_X^2 > 0$ and $S_Y^2 > 0$, there are unique values b and a for which $Q(a, b)$ always becomes minimal (the proof via partial differential equations is provided in the online material):

$$b = \frac{\text{Cov}(X, Y)}{S_X^2} = r_{XY}\frac{S_Y}{S_X} \quad \text{and} \quad a = M_Y - bM_X. \tag{11.6}$$

When plugging these values into the general equation of a straight line, the **regression equation** is:

$$\hat{Y} = r_{XY}\frac{S_Y}{S_X}X + M_Y - r_{XY}\frac{S_Y}{S_X}M_X$$

$$= r_{XY}\frac{S_Y}{S_X}(X - M_X) + M_Y. \tag{11.7}$$

Statisticians usually describe the prediction of $\hat{Y}$ by X, that is, $\hat{Y} = bX + a$ as the *regression of Y on X* (as in: Y is traced back to X).

With this information, we can determine the straight line that best represents any given data, at least in the sense of the least squares criterion. Two important *properties* apply to this straight line: First, if two variables are *linearly independent*, that is, if $r = 0$, we can see from Formula 11.7 that $\hat{Y} = M_Y$. In such a case, the regression line runs in parallel to the x-axis and intersects the y-axis at M_Y. In other words, the best prediction of any y_i value is M_Y. Second, in case $|r| = 1$, all empirical values lie exactly on the regression line.

11.3.2 Inferential Statistics of Simple Linear Regression

So far, we have considered how to determine b and a for the linear regression equation $\hat{Y} = bX + a$. In most cases, b and a will take values different from 0. The particular values, however, are again based on a sample, but we are actually interested in their values in the underlying population. The more relevant question is thus: Are the corresponding population parameters also different from 0?

Even if the regression parameters in the population are equal to 0, we are very likely to obtain empirical values different from 0. But only if, for example, the slope in the population differs from 0, it makes sense to consider b in predictions at all. The procedure for answering this question is the same as for the previous tests, and we will explain the procedure briefly for the slope parameter.

The slope b of the regression line is a sample statistic. At the population level, we call the slope the parameter β.[3] The hypotheses about β have a very similar form as those about ρ in Sect. 11.2.2:

$$H_0 : \beta = 0 \quad \text{and} \quad H_1 : \beta \neq 0.$$

The equation for determining b (Formula 11.6) already suggests a direct relationship to the correlation coefficient r. In fact, the test of these hypotheses about β is the same as the test of the correlation coefficient, and we use the same test statistic (see Formula 11.4):

$$t = \frac{r\sqrt{n-2}}{\sqrt{1-r^2}}.$$

Accordingly, the decision rule is also the same as in the case of the correlation. Of course, if a test performed on a correlation coefficient ρ is significant, the test performed on β from the corresponding simple linear regression will also be significant. The t-ratio is derived in more detail in Box 11.2.

In Depth 11.2: The t-Ratio as a Test Statistic for β

To determine the test statistic for β, we proceed as usual: We need a quantity that (1) comes with more extreme values, the more the data speak against the H_0 and (2) the distribution of which is known if the H_0 were true in the population. We start with the general form of the t-ratio (see Formula 5.5) and plug in the corresponding quantities of the regression:

$$t = \frac{T - \tau_0}{SE_T} = \frac{\hat{\beta} - 0}{SE_{\hat{\beta}}}. \tag{11.8}$$

Because $E(b) = \beta$, the slope b of the regression is an unbiased estimator for β. Determining the standard error of this estimator is more complicated, and it is:

$$SE_{\hat{\beta}} = \sqrt{\frac{\frac{S_Y^2(1-r_{XY}^2)}{n-2}}{S_X^2}}.$$

(continued)

---

[3] This β is different from, and must not be confused with, the β-error or the name of the effect β_k in factorial analysis of variance. The same is true for the so-called β-weights, which we will get to know later in this chapter (see Sect. 11.4.1).

We now substitute these estimates in Eq. 11.8. After some rearranging and by applying Eq. 11.6, we obtain:

$$t = \frac{b}{\sqrt{\frac{s_Y^2(1-r_{XY}^2)}{n-2}}} = \frac{b}{\frac{s_Y\sqrt{1-r_{XY}^2}}{s_X\sqrt{n-2}}} = b \cdot \frac{s_X\sqrt{n-2}}{s_Y\sqrt{1-r_{XY}^2}}$$

$$= b\underbrace{\frac{s_X}{s_Y}}_{=r_{XY}} \cdot \frac{\sqrt{n-2}}{\sqrt{1-r_{XY}^2}}.$$

Hence, it follows (see also Formula 11.4):

$$t = \frac{r\sqrt{n-2}}{\sqrt{1-r^2}}.$$

11.4 Outlook

Bivariate correlation and simple linear regression are the two simplest and most common approaches to testing correlation hypotheses, and we have seen that the general procedure for inferential statistics is identical to that for difference hypotheses. Finally, we briefly discuss two more complex procedures: multiple regression and partial correlation. For more information on correlation and regression analyses, we recommend Cohen et al. (2003).

11.4.1 Multiple Linear Regression

With simple linear regression (Sect. 11.3), we have introduced a way of dealing with *one* predictor variable X to predict a criterion variable Y. Often, however, a criterion can be predicted much better by using several predictors. In case of $m \geq 2$ predictors, we can utilize **multiple linear regression**. This approach generalizes the regression equation accordingly:

$$\hat{Y} = b_1X_1 + b_2X_2 + \dots b_mX_m + a.$$

The general procedure is identical to that for simple linear regression: the least squares method is used as the criterion to minimize the deviations of the predicted data from the empirical data. The calculation of the corresponding coefficients b_j and a is, however, more complicated and we leave this to appropriate computer programs.

> **In Depth 11.3: Variable Coding and Multicollinearity**
> When computing multiple regressions, it is useful to code all corresponding variables in a way that allows easy and straightforward interpretation. For binary predictor variables, coding with a distance of one unit is helpful (0 vs. 1 or -0.5 vs. 0.5) so that b-coefficients indicate the difference between both levels. In addition, using "centered" predictors, that is, a coding with a mean of 0 across all values, is recommended when the regression equation involves interactions between different predictors, while also avoiding predictor values of 0 (see Afshartous and Preston 2011). Finally, predictors should be as uncorrelated with each other as possible to allow meaningful estimation of regression coefficients (correlated predictors lead to so-called multicollinearity problems; see, e.g., Farrar and Glauber 1967).

The size of the coefficients b_j depends on the variance of the criterion and of the respective predictor X_j. Therefore, they cannot be interpreted to mean that a larger value b_j means "more influence" of the corresponding predictor X_j on the criterion Y. However, after an appropriate standardization, the resulting β-weights allow such an interpretation:

$$\beta_j = \frac{s_{X_j}}{s_Y} b_j. \tag{11.9}$$

11.4.2 Partial Correlation

Sometimes, the correlation between two variables X and Y depends on a third variable Z. In such a situation, the partial correlation can provide a remedy by removing the linear influence of Z. To illustrate the problem and the approach, let us first consider an example.

A magazine once reported that the starting salary of academics increases with study duration, and indeed there is a positive correlation between length of study and starting salary.[4] The left panel of Fig. 11.4 show fictitious values for both variables as a scatterplot of 18 persons. Assessing the whole data set indeed reveals a positive correlation and the plotted regression line has a positive slope.

In the right panel of Fig. 11.4, the data are split by the field of study. From this, we can immediately see that the correlation within each topic is in fact negative and the regression lines have a negative slope. The positive correlation across all data points only results

---

[4] This example comes from the German book by Krämer (2009, Chap. 14).

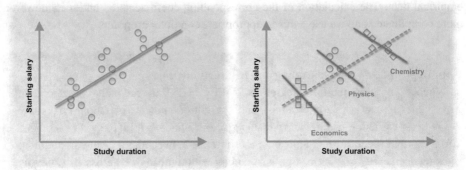

Fig. 11.4 Fictitious data on the relation between starting salary and study duration. The left panel shows the regression line across all data points; the right panel shows the data points broken down by field of study, and the solid lines are regression lines within each field

from the fact that (1) chemists generally had the longest time of study and (2) their starting salaries were also particularly high.

In this example, the relation between two variables depends on the level of a third variable: The relation between starting salary Y and study duration X depends on the field of study Z. If we were calculating the correlation for *constant levels* of Z separately (i.e., separately for each topic of study), we obtain a negative correlation in each case: the relationship of X and Y, if "the influence of Z is eliminated". Statisticians then say, the variable Z has been partialed out.

Mathematically, this problem is solved with the method of **partial correlation**; a method of finding the linear relationship between two variables X and Y after removing the (linear) relationship with a third variable Z. First, we determine the linear influence of Z on the variables X and Y by running the simple linear regressions of X and Y (as criteria) on Z (as the predictor):

$$\hat{X} = \frac{\text{Cov}(X, Z)}{S_Z^2}(Z - M_Z) + M_X$$

$$\hat{Y} = \frac{\text{Cov}(Y, Z)}{S_Z^2}(Z - M_Z) + M_Y.$$

Second, we can calculate the residuals

$$E_X = X - \hat{X} \quad \text{and} \quad E_Y = Y - \hat{Y}$$

that represent the variables X and Y with the linear influence of Z *removed* (the covariance of the residual variables and Z is indeed 0). Finally, the partial correlation of X and Y with respect to Z is simply the correlation of the two residual variables:

$$r_{XY \cdot Z} = r_{E_X E_Y} = \frac{r_{XY} - r_{XZ} r_{YZ}}{\sqrt{1 - r_{XZ}^2}\sqrt{1 - r_{YZ}^2}}.$$

When working with partial correlations, we implicitly assume that there is an equal correlation of X and Y under all levels of Z. If this is not true, there may also be situations in which the partial correlation becomes 0, although linear correlations exist for each level of Z.

The reason for this is that a partial correlation shifts, so to speak, the data points for all levels of Z and then calculates the correlation for the superimposed data. If the correlation is positive on half of the levels of Z, but negative on the other half, we can easily observe a zero correlation when running a partial correlation analysis.

11.4.3 Further Methods

Regression methods can also be used to analyze data that have a different structure than those considered so far, that is, data with one or more predictors and an interval-scaled criterion variable.

One important special case are **logistic regressions**, where a binary criterion is to be predicted (e.g., present vs. absent; true vs. false). A central score in such analyses is the so-called (logarithmic) odds ratio, that is, the ratio of the probabilities with which the two levels of the criterion occur. Despite high conceptual similarity with (multiple) linear regression, there are some notable peculiarities here, for instance, when it comes to interpreting the resulting regression coefficients. For more details, we refer to more specialized literature (Hosmer et al. 2013; for a compact introduction, see Tabachnick and Fidell 2012).

Furthermore, regression methods can also be applied to data with a hierarchical structure. This means that the data on one particular level are not completely independent from one another, but are instead structured into a higher-level variable (or multiple variables at multiple higher levels). A typical example is testing pupils from different classes, which in turn come from different schools. Such data are frequently encountered in, for example, educational psychology. Another example from cognitive psychology is when participants provide data for several different conditions (i.e., in within-subject designs). Should this hierarchical structure be taken into account, regression approaches can be used for data analyses as well.

Regression Coefficient Analysis (Lorch and Myers 1990), for instance, tackles this problem in two steps. The first step is calculating appropriate regressions for the lowest hierarchical level in each case (e.g., separate regressions over individual trials or responses of each participant). The second step then compares the coefficients between units of the next higher hierarchical level (for a practical introduction, see Pfister et al. 2013). The same idea underlies so-called **hierarchical linear models** (also: mixed-effects models; Baayen et al. 2008), except that here a simultaneous (and mathematically much more complex) estimation of regression coefficients takes place at all relevant levels (for an introduction, see also Bates et al. 2015).

11.5 Examples and Exercises

In this section, we analyze a data set with two variables: The number of books a person has read in the last year and their IQ as determined by an intelligence test. We want to find out whether there is a statistically significant relationship between the two variables (correlation) and whether IQ can be predicted from the number of books read (regression).

11.5.1 Correlation and Regression with R

The example data are stored in the file 11_data_correlation.dat available in the online material. We assume that the data are available as a data frame named data, which accordingly consists of two variables: books and IQ.

Determining the correlation of the two variables is very easy with the function cor():

```
cor(data$books, data$IQ)

0.6274089
```

This correlation is large following the terminology introduced in Sect. 11.2.1. Testing whether this correlation is also significantly different from 0 is possible with the function cor.test():

```
cor.test(data$books, data$IQ)

 Pearson's product-moment correlation
data: data$books and data$IQ
t = 3.4184, df = 18, p-value = 0.003064
```

According to the output, the correlation is significantly different from 0, $r = .63$, $t(18) = 3.42$, $p = .003$. The complete output contains further information about the confidence interval and the tested hypotheses (directional or non-directional). Several parameters can be specified when being passed as arguments to the cor.test()

function. The `cor_out()` function of the `schoRsch` package further allows to format the output. In addition, the function `ezCor()` from the `ez` package provides useful ways for calculating and visualizing correlations, especially when planning to compute separate bivariate correlations between several variables simultaneously.

Now we want to determine the regression line to predict IQ based on the amount of books read. This is possible with the function `lm()`, which requires the regression equation in R's modeling notation. For simple linear regression, the call is as follows:

```
# run the regression...
reg_result <- lm(data$IQ ~ data$books)

# ...and show the result
summary(reg_result)

Coefficients:
            Estimate Std. Error t value Pr(>|t|)
(Intercept) 89.6194     2.6405  33.941 < 2e-16 ***
data$books   0.5876     0.1719   3.418 0.00306 **

Residual standard error: 8.082 on 18 degs of freedom
Multiple R-squared: 0.3936, Adjusted R-squared: 0.36
F-statistic: 11.69 on 1 and 18 DF, p-value: 0.003064
```

The output provides statistics for both parameters of the regression line. The value for a is provided as the *intercept* and b according to the predictor variable's name, and the column *Estimate* presents the estimates of the parameters according to Formula 11.6, which are tested for significance automatically. In addition, R^2 is provided as a measure of how much of the total variability the regression line explains.

Other interesting functions that can be applied to `reg_result` are `coef()` to display only the regression coefficients (parameters), as well as `resid()` and `fitted()`, to display the residuals e_i or the predicted values $\hat{y}$. Furthermore, the function `lm()` can easily be called with more complex arguments, for example, to calculate multiple regression.

11.5.2 Correlation and Regression with SPSS

Exemplary data for calculating correlation and regression with SPSS can be found in the file `11_data_correlation.sav` in the online material. To calculate the correlation of the two variables `Books` and `IQ`, we use the menu

```
Analyze > Correlate > Bivariate...
```

There, we move both variables into the field *Variables* and after clicking on *OK*, we receive a correlation matrix in the output. This matrix includes several (inferential) statistical

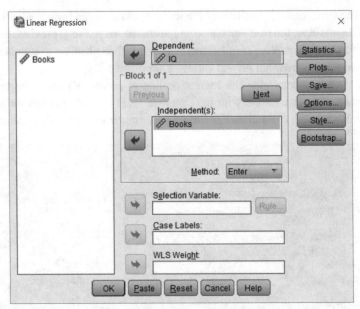

Fig. 11.5 Dialog box for running a linear regression with SPSS

parameters for each combination of the correlated variables: the correlation coefficient r, the p-value of the significance test, as well as the number of persons entered into the calculation (in our example there is of course only one meaningful combination, but this setup allows for correlating more than two variables easily and efficiently). For our example data, we obtain a significant positive correlation, $r = .63$, $p = .003$.[5]

Next we compute a simple linear regression with SPSS with the menu

`Analyze > Regression > Linear...`

In the dialog box (Fig. 11.5), we move the criterion (the dependent variable) IQ and the predictor (the independent variable) Books into the corresponding fields and confirm with *OK*.

The output offers a summary of the most important results in the table *Coefficients* (Fig. 11.6). This table shows (1) the intercept of the regression line on the y-axis (*Constant*; i.e., the value of a in Eq. 11.6) and (2) the slope of the regression line (*Books*; i.e., the value for b in Formula 11.6). The standardized β (see Formula 11.9) is also provided for the slope coefficient, since this function is also used to calculate multiple regressions. The table also provides the corresponding significance tests of the intercept and the slope

---

[5] In contrast to R, SPSS does not provide the t-value of the significance test as well. If required, it has to be calculated manually or taken from the output of a simple linear regression.

Coefficients[a]

Model		Unstandardized Coefficients		Standardized Coefficients	t	Sig.
		B	Std. Error	Beta		
1	(Constant)	89.619	2.640		33.941	.000
	Books	.588	.172	.627	3.418	.003

a. Dependent Variable: IQ

Fig. 11.6 Main output of a linear regression in SPSS

(each tested against a value of 0). In the example, we obtain a regression line with an intercept $a = 89.62$ which is significantly different from zero, $t(19) = 33.94$, $p < .001$. The slope of the regression line is $b = 0.59$ and is also significantly different from zero, $t(18) = 3.42$, $p = .003$.

Bayesian Alternatives

12

All inferential statistical procedures discussed in the preceding chapters belong to the group of so-called null hypothesis significance tests (often abbreviated as "NHST" in current discussions). Although the procedure of null hypothesis significance testing is widely used, far-reaching criticism of the underlying decision model is almost as old as the procedures themselves.

The recent past has seen an especially heated debate about the extent to which null hypothesis significance tests should be modified, supplemented by other procedures, or even completely replaced by these alternatives. In this chapter, we give an overview of so-called Bayesian procedures as the currently most prominent alternative to classical inferential statistics. In fact, numerous software solutions have been released in recent years that provide easy access to Bayesian alternatives for almost all common inferential statistical procedures. Whether these innovations actually provide added value is a matter that each researcher needs to decide for themselves. We will present arguments for and against the respective methods to facilitate this decision.

12.1   Two Concepts of Probability

As we have seen in previous chapters, classical inferential statistics employs a decision logic that does not aim to be correct for each single test. This would be an unattainable goal—instead, the aim is to make a correct decision in most cases across many investigations. The *concept of probability in classical inferential statistics* thus pertains to relative frequency: If the H_0 were true, then—on average—in 95 out of 100 cases the correct decision for the H_0 is made (assuming $\alpha = 0.05$), while the remaining five cases would yield a Type I error (see Chap. 4 and Chap. 7). If, on the other hand, the H_1 is true, then—on average—we will decide correctly in $(1 - \beta) \cdot 100\%$ of the cases, while committing

© Springer-Verlag GmbH Germany, part of Springer Nature 2023
M. Janczyk, R. Pfister, *Understanding Inferential Statistics*,
https://doi.org/10.1007/978-3-662-66786-6_12

a Type II error in the remaining cases. This notion of probabilities as relative frequencies over the course of many individual tests is also directly expressed in the p-value as one of the central statistics of null hypothesis significance tests, that is,

$$p = P(\text{data} | H_0).$$

The *concept of probability in Bayesian statistics*, by contrast, views probabilities as *beliefs*, that is, subjective probabilities of a particular hypothesis being true. In the context of scientific investigations, these beliefs are based on two aspects. First, on the collected data and, second, on prior assumptions about the general probability or plausibility of a hypothesis (so-called *priors*). Accordingly, Bayesian statistics highlights the following probability:

$$P(\text{hypothesis} | \text{data, assumptions}).$$

At first glance, Bayesian statistics thus seems to be geared more directly towards the question that we have previously answered only in an indirect way in the context of null hypothesis significance testing: the question of which hypothesis to believe in, given the available data. The seemingly close alignment of statistical analysis with the actual goal of an investigation is often seen as a major advantage of this method by advocates of Bayesian statistics (Dienes 2014; Kruschke 2010; Kruschke and Liddell 2018). Upon closer inspection though, the approach of Bayesian statistics is at least as indirect as is classical inferential statistics. We will briefly outline the basic idea of Bayesian methods in the following sections. It is based on **Bayes' theorem**, one of the central theorems of mathematical probability theory.

12.2   Bayes' Theorem

Bayes' theorem is named after a posthumous publication by Thomas Bayes (1701–1761) (for a historical treatise, see Barnard 1958). It describes the relationship between the two conditional probabilities $P(A|B)$ and $P(B|A)$, that is, the conditional probability of an event A given an event B, and the conditional probability of an event B given an event A, respectively. The probability $P(A \cap B)$, that is, the probability of the joint occurrence (intersection $A \cap B$) can be calculated in two ways:

$$P(A \cap B) = P(A|B) \cdot P(B)$$

and

$$P(A \cap B) = P(B|A) \cdot P(A)$$

We can see from these equations that $P(A|B) \cdot P(B) = P(B|A) \cdot P(A)$ and by rearrangement, we obtain Bayes' theorem as:

$$P(A|B) = \frac{P(B|A) \cdot P(A)}{P(B)} \qquad (12.1)$$

In Depth 12.1: Intuition and Clinical Diagnosis

Despite its simple mathematical makeup, Bayes' theorem often yields surprising results that challenge the intuition of many people. A particularly impressive example for such surprising results arises in the context of medical diagnosis (Eddy 1982; Gigerenzer and Hoffrage 1995).

Medical diagnoses resemble classical hypothesis tests in that they aim at deciding between competing hypotheses ("disease present" vs. "disease absent") based on empirical data. In this context, a medical examination is particularly helpful if it satisfies two quality criteria: sensitivity and specificity. High *sensitivity* means that an examination will likely recognize a disease if it is present—that is, high values for P(positive diagnosis|disease present) or short: $P(+|D)$. High *specificity* means that an examination will actually recognize a healthy person as such—that is, high values for P(negative diagnosis|disease absent) or short: $P(-|\neg D)$.

As an example for these concepts, let us consider a clinical method that is intended to provide indications of the presence of the autoimmune disease multiple sclerosis. The prevalence of this disease is about 2 in 1000 people (Kip et al. 2016) and we assume the method to have a sensitivity of 80% and a specificity of 95%. The question is: What is the probability that the disease is actually present if there is a positive test result, that is, $P(D|+)$?

Calculating this probability with Formula 12.1 further requires the probability $P(+)$ that a positive test result occurs in any given person. Making use of the law of total probability, this is calculated as

$$P(+) = P(+|D) \cdot P(D) + P(+|\neg D) \cdot P(\neg D)$$

$$= 0.8 \cdot 0.002 + (1 - 0.95) \cdot (1 - 0.002)$$

$$= 0.0515$$

From this follows:

$$P(D|+) = \frac{P(+|D) \cdot P(D)}{P(+)} = \frac{0.8 \cdot 0.002}{0.0515} = 0.0311$$

(continued)

The probability of actually having the disease in case of a (single) positive test result therefore is only about 3%, which clearly contradicts the intuition of many lay people, and also of many medical practitioners (Eddy 1982).

12.3   Bayesian Hypothesis Testing

In the context of empirical research, Bayes' theorem formalizes the relationship between hypotheses and data to decide between these hypotheses. To do this, we replace event A in Formula 12.1 with a hypothesis to be tested and event B with the collected data:

$$P(\text{hypothesis}|\text{data}) = \frac{P(\text{data}|\text{hypothesis}) \cdot P(\text{hypothesis})}{P(\text{data})} \tag{12.2}$$

At first glance, this allows for directly evaluating a hypothesis using empirical data, therefore suggesting direct implications for an initial research question. In the literature, the terms used in Eq. 12.2 are also referred to as:

- $P(\text{hypothesis}|\text{data})$: posterior probability
- $P(\text{data}|\text{hypothesis})$: likelihood
- $P(\text{hypothesis})$: prior probability (short: prior)
- $P(\text{data})$: marginal likelihood

If all terms to the right of the equal sign in Formula 12.2 were known, it would indeed be possible to calculate a probability for certain hypotheses based on the current data. Unfortunately, however, this is not straightforward at all, and we would like to highlight two critical limitations here.

The first restriction concerns the calculation of *likelihoods*, that is, of $P(\text{data}|$ hypothesis), because this calculation requires a specific hypothesis. As described in Sect. 4.1.2, null hypotheses tend to be specific, whereas the alternative hypothesis is only formulated non-specifically in many situations. This is the reason why classical null hypothesis significance tests calculate the p-value assuming that the null hypothesis is true and then base the decisions on this value (see Chap. 4; in fact, in Bayesian terminology, a classical null hypothesis test is equivalent to computing a likelihood for the null hypothesis). A necessary prerequisite for conducting any Bayesian hypothesis test is thus to formulate a specific alternative hypothesis.[1]

---

[1] Some popular methods for computing Bayesian hypothesis tests circumvent this limitation by drawing on a special probability distribution called the Cauchy distribution (e.g., Rouder et al. 2009). The mathematical details of this approach are not trivial and, in particular, it also involves an estimate

The second limitation concerns the estimation of the *prior probability* and the *marginal likelihood*. Especially the latter term cannot be determined easily in most settings (or only at great computational expense). However, if we formulate Formula 12.2 for two hypotheses, H_0 and H_1 for example, and then divide both terms, the two marginal likelihoods cancel each other in the resulting ratio:

$$\underbrace{\frac{P(H_0|\text{data})}{P(H_1|\text{data})}}_{=\text{posterior odds ratio}} = \frac{\frac{P(\text{data}|H_0)\cdot P(H_0)}{P(\text{data})}}{\frac{P(\text{data}|H_1)\cdot P(H_1)}{P(\text{data})}} = \underbrace{\frac{P(\text{data}|H_0)}{P(\text{data}|H_1)}}_{=\text{Bayes Factor}} \cdot \underbrace{\frac{P(H_0)}{P(H_1)}}_{=\text{prior odds ratio}}$$

The ratio of two *likelihoods* that indicates which of two competing hypotheses more correctly reflects the available data is also called the **Bayes Factor** (BF):

$$\text{BF}_{01} = \frac{P(\text{data}|H_0)}{P(\text{data}|H_1)} = \frac{P(H_0|\text{data})}{P(H_1|\text{data})} \cdot \frac{P(H_1)}{P(H_0)}. \tag{12.3}$$

The index 01 indicates which hypothesis forms the numerator (the first digit) and the denominator (the second digit) of the Bayes Factor. For further simplification, Bayesians often assume $P(H_0) = P(H_1)$ (Rouder et al. 2009). This common, but not necessarily valid assumption, renders the *prior odds ratio* exactly 1, and the Bayes Factor can then be taken to indicate how much more likely one hypothesis is relative to the other (i.e., the *posterior odds ratio*).

The Bayes Factor is the central result of a Bayesian hypothesis test, and different Bayesian hypothesis tests have recently been developed for all common methods of classical inferential statistics (see also Sect. 12.5).[2] There also are numerous proposals in the literature on how to interpret certain values of Bayes Factors (Dienes 2016; Jeffreys 1961; Kass and Raftery 1995; Schönbrodt et al. 2017; Wetzels et al. 2011). Table 12.1 lists a common classification that combines the proposals of Jeffreys (1961) and Kass and Raftery (1995).

The values listed in Table 12.1 apply only to evidence for the model that is included in the numerator of Formula 12.3. Bayes Factors with a value of $\text{BF}_{01} > 1$ would be evidence

---

of the effect size to be expected under the alternative hypothesis, which tends to be hidden behind various default values that are set automatically in common software packages.

[2] In addition to Bayes Factors, Bayesian statistics also provide a range of other measures with unique properties, such as the *Bayesian Information Criterion* (*BIC;* e.g., Raftery 1995). However, Bayes Factors currently represent the most popular method in the social and behavioral sciences, so that we focus on this method here.

Table 12.1 Interpretation of Bayes Factors, based on the classifications of Jeffreys (1961) and Kass and Raftery (1995). The scale only considers evidence for the model that is listed in the numerator of the Bayes Factor

Bayes factor	Evidence
1–3	Anecdotal (i.e., negligible)
3–10	Substantial
10–30	Strong
30–100	Very strong
> 100	Extreme

for the H_0, while $BF_{01} < 1$ would be evidence for the H_1. However, BF_{01} and BF_{10} are interrelated:

$$BF_{01} = \frac{1}{BF_{10}}.$$

12.4 Evaluation of Bayesian Methods

The current discussion in psychological research methods as well as among applied statisticians is characterized by increasing mistrust in methods from classical inferential statistics, which are often blamed for problems such as lacking replicability of empirical results (e.g., Wagenmakers 2007; Wasserstein and Lazar 2016; Wasserstein et al. 2019). In this context, proponents of Bayesian statistics usually argue that Bayesian methods offer a genuinely superior approach to the analysis of empirical data (Dienes 2014; Kruschke 2010; Kruschke and Liddell 2018).

Whether one decides to share this view, however, is a decision that any researcher should make for themselves. It is true that Bayesian methods have some advantages over classical methods, but these advantages come at the expense of accepting other limitations and making further assumptions, some of which are not always obvious (see also Tendeiro and Kiers 2019). Bayesian methods are also far less standardized than classical methods, so that there is currently less consensus on how to calculate and especially on how to interpret the resulting Bayes Factors. This is especially evident from the large number of alternatives available for calculating a simple t-test (see Sect. 12.5), but also from the numerous proposals for interpreting the value of a Bayes Factor. For example, a Bayes Factor of $BF_{10} = 3$ is regarded by many authors as substantial evidence for the alternative hypothesis (e.g., Dienes 2016), while other authors only consider a Bayes Factor from $BF_{10} = 6$ or $BF_{10} = 10$ as substantial evidence for the alternative hypothesis (both latter suggestions can be found in Schönbrodt et al. 2017).

Furthermore, in light of the common argument of a qualitative difference between classical methods and their Bayesian alternatives, it should be noted that both variants

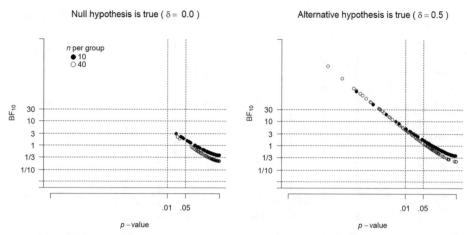

Fig. 12.1 Relation of p-values and Bayes Factors (BF_{10}; large values are evidence for the alternative hypothesis). Data points show the p-value and the BF_{10} for each of 100 comparisons of two samples with a size of $n = 10$ or $n = 40$ persons, respectively, using a classical t-test for independent samples and a corresponding Bayesian alternative, respectively. The simulation underlying the left panel of the figure assumes the null hypothesis to be true, whereas the simulation underlying the right panel assumes an effect of $\delta = 0.5$ between the populations. For illustrative purposes, p-values and Bayes Factors are plotted in a logarithmic scale

often lead to very similar conclusion. Decisions based on Bayes Factors thus mirror those based on p-values, albeit being slightly more conservative. This is suggested, for example, by data from a large-scale comparative study (Wetzels et al. 2011). Figure 12.1 shows the strength of this relationship using simulated data. Due to this tight relation, and because of the lack of a consensus on the exact interpretation of Bayes Factors, we do not see a compelling reason to generally prefer Bayesian procedures over classical null hypothesis tests at present.

   A possible advantage of Bayesian methods might arise if a study aims to gather evidence in favor of the null hypothesis, however. Classical inferential statistics can do this only to a limited extent (see Sect. 7.5 and Box 7.3), whereas Bayesian statistics explicitly provide the possibility of supplying evidence for the null hypothesis over the alternative hypothesis. But why does classical inferential statistics come to its limit here? To answer this question, it is helpful to consider how p-values are distributed if either the H_1 or the H_0 is true. We can illustrate this again with a set of simulations (see Fig. 12.2). For these simulations, we have either assumed that the null hypothesis is true (left panel of Fig. 12.2) or that the alternative hypothesis is true with $\delta = 0.5$ (right panel of Fig. 12.2). We then generated 100 pairs of independent samples in each case and compared them with a t-test. The sample sizes (per group) were either 2, 10, 20, 40, 60, 80, or 100. The small dots in Fig. 12.2 represent individual p-values; the large dots are the means of these individual p-values. In case of the alternative hypothesis, we see what would also be expected in light of power analyses: as sample size increases, the p-values tend to become smaller, with the

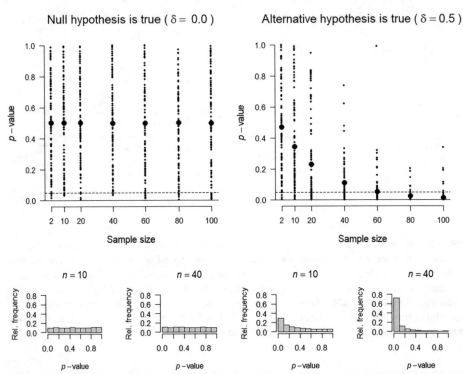

Fig. 12.2 Results of a simulation illustrating the distribution of p-values in case the null hypothesis is true (left panel) and in case the alternative hypothesis is true with $\delta = 0.5$ (right panel). The upper panels represent the p-values of 100 t-tests each for independent samples (small dots) and their mean (large dots) for different sample sizes. The bar plots in the lower panels show the relative frequencies of p-values for two exemplary sample sizes of 10,000 tests each

majority of the p-values being in the lower range. This pattern becomes even clearer in the two bar plots in the inset of the right panel: Here we have calculated the p-values of 10,000 t-tests and plotted their relative frequencies for the exemplary sample sizes $n = 10$ and $n = 40$. Small p-values occur more frequently than large p-values, and this pattern is more pronounced for larger compared to small sample sizes.

If the null hypothesis is true, however, the p-values behave completely differently. Indeed, in this case, all p-values are equally likely, and this is also independent of the sample size. In contrast to when the alternative hypothesis is true, the p-values also do not become smaller or larger on average, but remain at the same level for all sample sizes. The reason for the equal distribution of the p-values under the null hypothesis is—somewhat simplified—its own definition: The probability of $p \leq 0.05$ is exactly 0.05, that of $p \leq 0.10$ is exactly 0.10, etc (for more information, see Hung et al. 1997, or Simmons et al. 2011, and Ulrich and Miller 2018). Bayes Factors, on the other hand, behave more intuitively here, because as sample sizes increase, BF_{10} tends to become smaller and BF_{01} tends to become larger (Rouder et al. 2009).

Thus, if a research question aims at gathering evidence in favor of the null hypothesis, that is, if evidence for the absence of an effect is to be collected rather than merely attesting to the absence of evidence for that effect, Bayes statistics can be a meaningful tool. Of course, the criticism of heterogeneous evaluation guidelines mentioned above applies here as well; and even in this area of application, classical methods and Bayesian alternatives often produce consistent results (see Fig. 12.1).

Overall, then, it appears that Bayesian procedures provide a possible alternative to classical null hypothesis significance tests, yet they do not necessarily lead to more valid conclusions. In our view, the same assessment applies to other alternative approaches (such as the so-called "new statistics"; Cumming 2014). Every statistical procedure comes with its own sources of errors and peculiarities, and wrong decisions can never be ruled out with certainty in empirical investigations. We still believe that the current discussion on limitations and pitfalls of certain statistical procedures is helpful. After all, competently applying and interpreting the result of any statistical procedure is only possible if one is aware of precisely these limitations and pitfalls. Increasing sensitization of the relevant users—students, researchers, and teachers—is already becoming apparent, and can help to increase the reliability and credibility of empirical research results.

12.5 Examples and Exercises

Numerous solutions for a computational implementation of Bayesian procedures have been proposed in the last 10 years. This development has produced various online calculators (e.g., Dienes 2014), R packages (in particular, the `BayesFactor` package; Morey et al. 2019), and specialized software environments such as the JASP program (JASP Team 2018). Recent versions of SPSS also provide selected Bayesian methods (version 25 and above). The particular methods used to calculate Bayes Factors can differ greatly between different programs, and even different versions of the same program sometimes produce notably diverging results. It is therefore important to be mindful of these differences when choosing a suitable program, and to document the program's version, the corresponding settings, as well as the *prior probability* (or corresponding scale parameters). Finally, the available software solutions differ with respect to the data required: While some programs compute Bayes Factors via a direct transformation of a t- or F-value and provide no or only indirect options for specifying the expected effect size, other procedures assume a much more precise specification of the alternative hypothesis.

In the following, we will give examples of how to implement a t-test and a two-way analysis of variance (ANOVA) with the R package `BayesFactor` (version 0.9.12-4.2), followed by analogous examples for SPSS and JASP, respectively. It should be noted that even this limited selection of programs leads to numerically different results due to the lack of standardized methods.

12.5.1 Bayesian Hypothesis Tests with R

- **Example 1:** Bayesian t-test for two independent samples. As for the classical t-test from Chap. 5, we again use data on the yield of two fictitious areas that the Guinness Brewery might use to grow hop (Table 5.1). We assume that the data have been read as described in Chap. 5 and made available via the `attach()` function. In addition, the package `BayesFactor` must be installed and loaded to make the relevant function `ttestBF()` available:[3]

```
# load package
library(BayesFactor)
# run Bayesian t-test
ttestBF(x = yield[area == 1],
        y = yield[area == 2])
```

The output provides an estimate of the BF_{10}, which, like the classical t-test from Chap. 5. argues for a strong difference between the two growing areas ($BF_{10} = 10.02$):

```
Bayes factor analysis
--------------
[1] Alt., r=0.707 : 10.02015 ±0%

Against denominator:
  Null, mu1-mu2 = 0
---
Bayes factor type: BFindepSample, JZS
```

- **Example 2:** Bayesian ANOVA. We will now compute a Bayesian alternative to the classical two-way ANOVA from Chap. 9 using the package `BayesFactor` (for the corresponding data, see Table 8.2). Again, we ask whether memory performance (measured by the number of recalled words) is affected by sleep deprivation in younger and older adults. As in Chap. 9, we assume that the data have been read and that all relevant variables have been factorized (see Sect. 9.4.1). Now we can load the package

---

[3] In addition to `ttestBF()`, the `BayesFactor` package also provides the `ttest.tstat()` function, which estimates the Bayes Factor using the t-value of a classical test. The use of this function (as well as various additional arguments of the `ttestBF()` function) is described in the online material. For the available data, the function `ttest.tstat()` returns a result of $BF_{10} = 16.41$, which is obviously not the same as the output of the `ttestBF()` function.

BayesFactor and use the function `anovaBF()`, passing the data and the model in the modeling language of R (see Sect. 8.6.1 and the online material for Chaps. 8 and 9):

```
library(BayesFactor)
anovaBF(recalled_words ~ sleep_deprivation * age_group,
        data = data)
```

One possible result of this function is given below. Note that the function uses an iterative algorithm that produces (slightly) different results each time it is called, and one particular result is thus not necessarily reproducible (see also Pfister 2021):

```
Bayes factor analysis
--------------
[1] sleep_deprivation                    : 144.2842 ±0%
[2] age_group                            : 2.180258 ±0%
[3] sleep_deprivation + age_group        : 1586.721 ±0.94%
[4] sleep_deprivation + age_group +
        sleep_deprivation:age_group : 3234.07  ±1.38%

Against denominator:
   Intercept only
```

Each row of the output provides a Bayes Factor for the comparison of the specified model—defined via the factors included into the model equation—with the null model, which only consists of the grand mean of the data (colons indicate an interaction of two or more factors).

If we wanted to compare two models with each other rather than with the null model, we can make use of the fact that Bayes Factors are *ratios* of likelihoods. If the Bayes Factors of two models are put in relation to each other, identical terms cancel each other out (in this case: the null model), so that the ratio of two Bayes Factors in the output corresponds to the Bayes Factor for the corresponding model comparison. In our example, we see that Bayesian ANOVA does not provide substantial, but only anecdotal, evidence for the interaction of sleep deprivation and age group, because the Bayes Factor for the comparison of the third and fourth models in the output is $BF_{10} = \frac{3234.07}{1586.72} = 1.97$. This demonstrates the conservative nature of Bayesian methods mentioned in Sect. 12.4.

12.5.2 Bayesian Hypothesis Tests with SPSS and JASP

- **Example 1:** Bayesian *t*-tests for two independent samples. As for the classical *t*-test from Chap. 5, we again use data on the yield of two fictitious areas that the Guinness

Group Statistics

	Area	N	Mean	Std. Deviation	Std. Error Mean
Yield	= 1	10	35.20	5.245	1.659
	= 2	10	26.90	6.027	1.906

Bayes Factor Independent Sample Test (Method = Rouder)[a]

	Mean Difference	Pooled Std. Error Difference	Bayes Factor[b]	t	df	Sig.(2-tailed)
Yield	-8.30	2.527	.092	-3.285	18	.004

a. Assumes unequal variance between groups.

b. Bayes factor: Null versus alternative hypothesis.

Fig. 12.3 SPSS output for the Bayesian variant of the t-test for independent samples (available from SPSS 25 onward). The BF_{01} is provided by default

Brewery might use to grow hop (Table 5.3). We assume that the data were read as described in Chap. 5. We then select the dialog box

```
Analyze > Bayesian Statistics > Independent Samples Normal
```

and add the variable `Area` to the field *Grouping Variable*. The groups are then defined via *Define Groups...* by specifying the coding of the groups (1 or 2). As for the classic t-test, we add the variable `Yield` to the field *Test Variable(s)* and request Bayes Factors under *Bayesian Analysis*. Clicking *OK* starts the calculation and opens the output (Fig. 12.3).

The resulting Bayes Factor is $BF_{01} = 0.092$ or $BF_{10} = \frac{1}{BF_{01}} = 10.87$. Mirroring the classical t-test from Chap. 5, this result indicates a large difference between the two growing areas.[4]

- **Example 2:** Bayesian ANOVA. The current version of SPSS (27) only implements one-way ANOVA, and does not support factorial or repeated-measures designs. We therefore recommend the freely available program JASP (JASP Team 2018) for calculating Bayesian alternatives, which offers a comparable user interface.

---

[4] The Bayes Factors computed by SPSS and R differ slightly (R: $BF_{10} = 10.02$, SPSS: $BF_{10} = \frac{1}{BF_{01}} = 10.87$). This happens because SPSS uses a scaling parameter of 1 by default (options to change this default value are available in the *Priors...* menu, but do not seem to affect the calculation in any available version of SPSS—such as version 25.0.0). Both calculations do match if passing the parameter `rscale = 1` to the function `ttestBF()` of the R-package `BayesFactor` (version 0.9.12-4).

We will thus use JASP to compute a Bayesian alternative to the classical two-way ANOVA from Chap. 9. Again, we ask whether memory performance (measured by the number of recalled words) is affected by sleep deprivation in younger and older adults. The corresponding data from Table 8.2 must first be pre-processed as in Chap. 9 and saved as a .csv file (a corresponding file is available in the online material). Then we select the menu

```
ANOVA > Bayesian ANOVA
```

and insert the variable Recalled_Words into the field *Dependent Variable*, and the two variables Sleep_Deprivation and Age_Group into the field *Fixed Factors*. A click on *OK* finishes the input and opens the output.

One possible result of this function is shown in Fig. 12.4. Note that the function uses an iterative algorithm that produces (slightly) different results each time it is called, so each actual result is not necessarily reproducible (see also Pfister 2021). Each line of the output contains a Bayes Factor for the comparison of the specified model with the null model, which only consists of the grand mean of the data (asterisks indicate an interaction of two or more factors).

If we want to compare two models, we exploit the fact that Bayes Factors are *ratios* of likelihoods. If the Bayes Factors of two models are set in relation to each other, identical terms are canceled out (in this case: the null model), so that the ratio of two Bayes Factors in the output corresponds to the Bayes Factor for the corresponding model comparison. Here, we see that Bayesian ANOVA does not provide substantial, but only anecdotal evidence for the interaction of sleep deprivation and age group,

Model Comparison - Recalled_Words

Models	P(M)	P(M|data)	BF_M	BF_{10}	error %
Null model	0.2	1.944e-4	7.779e-4	1.000	
Sleep_Deprivation	0.2	0.028	0.115	144.284	0.001
Age_Group	0.2	4.239e-4	0.002	2.180	7.340e-4
Sleep_Deprivation + Age_Group	0.2	0.327	1.943	1681.670	2.456
Sleep_Deprivation + Age_Group + Sleep_Deprivation ∗ Age_Group	0.2	0.644	7.247	3313.824	3.346

Fig. 12.4 JASP output for a Bayesian two-way ANOVA. Bayes factors of each model are calculated relative to the null model (first row). Plus signs indicate models that assume additive combinations of two or more factors, asterisks indicate interactions

Model Comparison - Recalled_Words

Models	P(M)	P(M|data)	BF $_M$	BF $_{10}$	error %
Null model (incl. Sleep_Deprivation, Age_Group)	0.5	0.337	0.509	1.000	
Sleep_Deprivation * Age_Group	0.5	0.663	1.966	1.966	1.433

Note. All models include Sleep_Deprivation, Age_Group.

Fig. 12.5 JASP output of a Bayesian two-way ANOVA with the two main effects added to the null model. The resulting Bayes Factor of 1.97 for the interaction corresponds to the comparison of the main effect model with the saturated model from Fig. 12.4, that is, the model that includes all possible main effects and interactions of the factors used

because the Bayes Factor for the comparison of the last and second-to-last model in the output is $BF_{10} = \frac{3313.82}{1681.67} = 1.97$ (the same result is obtained when we add the two main effects to the null model under *Model*; see Fig. 12.5). This shows the conservative nature of Bayesian methods mentioned in Sect. 12.4.

Concluding Remarks

13

The preceding chapters of this book have covered several test procedures from the realm of inferential statistics. We have focused mainly on tests for hypotheses about differences between population parameters, including the various t-tests and analyses of variance. This was followed by a brief take on hypotheses about relations or dependencies, with a focus on correlation and regression.

These procedures allow to evaluate a wide variety of data sets and thus to statistically validate substantive hypotheses in many research fields. It goes without saying that the toolbox of inferential statistics offers many more tests than we have covered here. Against this background, however, it is crucial to remember that all inferential tests follow the same general procedure. Once you have understood this procedure, you will have the necessary tools to perform any statistical test correctly and to interpret its result. We therefore summarize the most important points here again:

1. Each test begins with transforming a substantive hypothesis into statistical hypotheses. The latter can refer to any population parameter (e.g., μ, σ^2, or ρ) and are formulated as a pair of a null hypothesis H_0 and an alternative hypothesis H_1. The H_0 usually includes the case that there is no difference or relation in the population.
2. Because we cannot measure the population parameter directly in most cases, we have to rely on samples that we draw from the population. These samples allow us to calculate estimators of the parameter of interest (e.g., M, $\hat{S}^2$, or r).
3. We then have to compute a suitable test statistic based on these estimators. Any test statistic has to fulfill at least two requirements: It should (1) take more extreme values the more the data speak against the H_0, and (2) its distribution should be known under the assumption that the H_0 is true. (More precisely, the distribution of a random variable that assigns the test statistic to the sample(s) in question.)

© Springer-Verlag GmbH Germany, part of Springer Nature 2023
M. Janczyk, R. Pfister, *Understanding Inferential Statistics*,
https://doi.org/10.1007/978-3-662-66786-6_13

4. The H_0 is at the core of this procedure because—unlike the H_1—it is usually formulated as a specific hypothesis and thus allows for determining the distribution (or probability density function) of the test statistic. With this distribution at hand, we can determine probabilities for observing values in a certain value range.
5. Finally, we make a simple decision between the two hypotheses: If the observed (or more extreme) data are sufficiently unlikely ($p \leq \alpha$) when assuming the H_0 to be true, we decide in favor of the H_1. If this is not the case, then we retain the H_0. By convention, the significance level is set to $\alpha = .05$ in most studies.

On closer inspection, the only difference between different test procedures is which test statistic is calculated from the empirical data and, thus, which distribution is used to inform the decision. This applies similarly to a large number of inferential statistical procedures that we have not covered in this book, though an informed understanding of the above procedure will allow for adopting any of these procedures easily. Crucially, what all these test procedures have in common is that they allow us to make statements that go beyond the data at hand—that is, statements that can have precisely the general character scientists should aim for in their work.

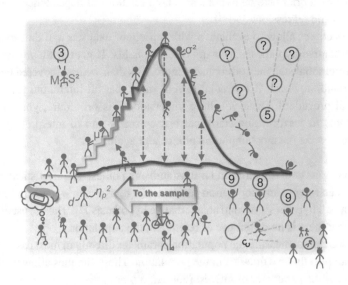

References

Afshartous, D., & Preston, R. A. (2011). Key results of interaction models with centering. *Journal of Statistics Education, 19*, 1–24.

APA. (2020). *Publication manual of the American Psychological Association* (7th ed.). APA.

Baayen, R. H., Davidson, D. J., & Bates, D. M. (2008). Mixed-effects modeling with crossed random effects for subjects and items. *Journal of Memory and Language, 59*, 390–412.

Baguley, T. (2012). Calculating and graphing within-subjects confidence intervals. *Behavior Research Methods, 44*, 158–175.

Bakeman, R., & McArthur, D. (1996). Picturing repeated measures: Comments on Loftus, Morrison, and others. *Behavior Research Methods, Instruments, & Computers, 28*, 584–589.

Barnard, G. A. (1958). Studies in the history of probability and statistics: IX. Thomas Bayes's essay towards solving a problem in the doctrine of chances. *Biometrika, 45*, 293–295.

Bates, D., Mächler, M., Bolker, B., & Walker, S. (2015). Fitting linear mixed-effects models using lme4. *Journal of Statistical Software, 67*, 1–48.

Belia, S., Fidler, F., Williams, J., & Cumming, G. (2005). Researchers misunderstand confidence intervals and standard error bars. *Psychological Methods, 10*, 389–396.

Bennett, C. M., Baird, A. A., Miller, M. B., & Wolford, G. L. (2011). Neural correlates of interspecies perspective taking in the post-mortem Atlantic Salmon: An argument for proper multiple comparisons corrections. *Journal of Serendipitous and Unexpected Results, 1*, 1–5.

Bortz, J. (2005). *Statistik für Human- und Sozialwissenschaftler*. Springer.

Bortz, J., & Schuster, C. (2010). *Statistik für Human- und Sozialwissenschaftler*. Springer.

Box, G. E. P. (1954). Some theorems on quadratic forms applied in the study of analysis of variance problems, I. Effect of inequality of variance in the one-way classification. *Annals of Mathematical Statistics, 25*, 290–302.

Cantor, G. N. (1956). A note on a methodological error commonly committed in medical and psychological research. *American Journal of Mental Deficiency, 61*, 17–18.

Cohen, J. (1988). *Statistical power analysis for the behavioral sciences.* (2nd ed.). Erlbaum.

Cohen, J. (1990). Things I have learned (so far). *American Psychologist, 45*, 1304–1312.

Cohen, J., Cohen, P., West, S. G., & Aiken, L. S. (2003). *Applied multiple regression/correlation analysis for the behavioral sciences* (3rd ed.). Erlbaum.

Cousineau, D. (2005). Confidence intervals in withinsubject designs: A simpler solution to Loftus and Masson's method. *Tutorials in Quantitative Methods for Psychology, 1*, 42–45.

Cousineau, D. (2017). Varieties of confidence intervals. *Advances in Cognitive Psychology, 13*, 140–155.

© Springer-Verlag GmbH Germany, part of Springer Nature 2023
M. Janczyk, R. Pfister, *Understanding Inferential Statistics*,
https://doi.org/10.1007/978-3-662-66786-6

Cousineau, D. (2019). Correlation-adjusted standard errors and confidence intervals for within-subject designs: A simple multiplicative approach. *The Quantitative Methods for Psychology, 15*(3), 226–241.

Crossman, E. R. F. W. (1959). A theory of the acquisition of speed-skill. *Ergonomics, 2*, 153–166.

Cumming, G. (2014). The new statistics: Why and how. *Psychological Science, 25*, 7–29.

Cumming, G., & Finch, S. (2005). Inference by eye. Confidence intervals and how to read pictures of data. *American Psychologist, 60*, 170–180.

de Vries, A., & Meys, J. (2012). *R for dummies*. John Wiley & Sons.

DGPs. (2007). *Richtlinien zur Manuskriptgestaltung [Guidelines for manuscript preparation]* (3rd ed.). Hogrefe.

Diaz-Bone, R., & Künemund, H. (2003). *Einführung in die binäre logistische Regression.* Mitteilungen aus dem Schwerpunktbereich Methodenlehre (Heft Nr. 56).

Dienes, Z. (2014). Using Bayes to get the most out of non-significant results. *Frontiers in Psychology, 5*, 781.

Dienes, Z. (2016). How Bayes factors change scientific practice. *Journal of Mathematical Psychology, 72*, 78–89.

Dracup, C. (2005). Confidence intervals. In B. S. Everitt & D. C. Howell (Eds.), *Encyclopedia of statistics in behavioral science* (Vol. 1, pp. 366–375). John Wiley & Sons.

Dunlap, W. P., Cortina, J. M., Vaslow, J. B., & Burke, M. J. (1996). Meta-analysis of experiments with matched groups or repeated measures designs. *Psychological Methods, 1*, 170–177.

Eddy, D. M. (1982). Probabilistic reasoning in clinical medicine: Problems and opportunities. In D. Kahneman, P. Slovic, & A. Tversky (Eds.), *Judgment under uncertainty: Heuristics and biases* (pp. 249–267). Cambridge University Press.

Eid, M., Gollwitzer, M., & Schmitt, M. (2010). *Statistik und Forschungsmethoden [Statistics and research methods]*. Beltz.

Ellis, P. D. (2010). *The essential guide to effect sizes: Statistical power, meta-analysis, and the interpretation of research results*. Cambridge University Press.

Farrar, D. E., & Glauber, R. R. (1967). Multicollinearity in regression analysis: The problem revisited. *The Review of Economic and Statistics, 49*, 92–107.

Faul, F., Erdfelder, E., Lang, A.-G., & Buchner, A. (2007). G*Power 3: A flexible statistical power analysis program for the social, behavioral, and biomedical sciences. *Behavior Research Methods, 39*, 175–191.

Fienberg, S. E. (1992). A brief history of statistics in three and one-half chapters: A review essay. *Statistical Science, 7*, 208–225.

Fisher, R. A. (1935). *The design of experiments*. Oliver & Boyd.

Fitts, P. M., & Posner, M. I. (1967). *Human performance*. Prentice-Hall.

Francis, G., Tanzman, J., & Matthews, W. (2014). Excess success for psychology articles in the journal Science. *PLoS One, 9*, e114255.

Franz, V., & Loftus, G. (2012). Standard errors and confidence intervals in within-subjects designs: Generalizing Loftus and Masson (1994) and avoiding the biases of alternative accounts. *Psychonomic Bulletin & Review, 19*, 395–404.

Gigerenzer, G., & Hoffrage, U. (1995). How to improve Bayesian reasoning without instruction: Frequency formats. *Psychological Review, 102*, 684–704.

Gigerenzer, G., & Murray, D. J. (1987). *Cognition as intuitive statistics*. Erlbaum.

Goulet-Pelletier, J. C., & Cousineau, D. (2018). A review of effect sizes and their confidence intervals, Part I: The Cohen's *d* family. *The Quantitative Methods for Psychology, 14*, 242–265.

Greenhouse, S., & Geisser, S. (1959). On methods in the analysis of profile data. *Psychometrika, 24*, 95–112.

Hollander, M., Wolfe, D. A., & Chicken, E. (2014). *Nonparametric statistical methods.* John Wiley & Sons.

Hosmer, D. W., Jr., Lemeshow, S., & Sturdivant, R. X. (2013). *Applied logistic regression.* John Wiley & Sons.

Howell, D. C, (2017). *Fundamental statistics for the behavioral sciences* (9th ed.). Cengage Learning.

Hubbard, R. (2011). The widespread misinterpretation of p-values as error probabilities. *Journal of Applied Statistics, 38,* 2617–2626.

Hung, H. J., O'Neill, R. T., Bauer, P., & Kohne, K. (1997). The behavior of the p-value when the alternative hypothesis is true. *Biometrics, 53,* 11–22.

Iacobucci, D. (1995). Analysis of variance for unbalanced data. *Marketing Theory and Applications, 6,* 337–343.

JASP Team. (2018). JASP (version 0.10.0) [Computer software]. https://jasp-stats.org/

Janssen, J., & Laatz, W. (2010). *Statistische Datenanalyse mit SPSS* (7th ed.). Springer.

Jeffreys, H. (1961). *Theories of probability* (3rd ed.). Oxford University Press.

Kass, E. E., & Raftery, A. E. (1995). Bayes factors. *Journal of the American Statistical Association, 90,* 773–795.

Keppel, G., & Wickens, T. D. (2004). *Design and analysis. A researcher's handbook.* Pearson.

Kip, M., Zimmermann, A., & Bleß, H.-H., (2016). Epidemiologie der Multiplen Sklerose. In M. Kip, T. Schönfelder, & H.-H. Bleß (Eds.), *Weißbuch Multiple Sklerose* (pp. 13–21). Springer.

Krämer, W. (2009). *So lügt man mit Statistik* (12th ed.). Piper.

Kruschke, J. K. (2010). What to believe: Bayesian methods for data analysis. *Trends in Cognitive Sciences, 14,* 293–300.

Kruschke, J. K., & Liddell, T. M. (2018). The Bayesian new statistics: Hypothesis testing, estimation, meta-analysis, and power analysis from a Bayesian perspective. *Psychonomic Bulletin & Review, 25,* 178–206.

Kubinger, K. D., Rasch, D., & Moder, K. (2009). Zur Legende der Voraussetzungen des t-Tests für unabhängige Stichproben. *Psychologische Rundschau, 60,* 26–27.

Lakens, D. (2013). Calculating and reporting effect sizes to facilitate cumulative science: A practical primer for t-tests and ANOVAs. *Frontiers in Psychology, 4,* 863.

Lakens, D. (2017). Equivalence tests: A practical primer for t tests, correlations, and meta-analyses. *Social Psychological and Personality Science, 8,* 355–362.

Lane, D. M. (2016). The assumption of sphericity in repeated-measures designs: What it means and what to do when it is violated. *The Quantitative Methods for Psychology, 12,* 114–122.

Langenberg, B., Janczyk, M., Koob, V., Kliegl, R., & Mayer, A. (2022). A tutorial on using the paired t test for power calculations in repeated measures ANOVA with interactions. *Behavior Research Methods.*

Lawrence, M. A. (2016). ez: Easy analysis and visualization of factorial experiments (Version 4.4-0) [Computer software]. https://CRAN.R-project.org/package=ez

Levene, H. (1960). Robust tests for equality of variances. In S. G. Ghurye, W. Hoeffding, W. G., & Madow H. B. Mann (Eds.), *Contributions to probability and statistics: Essays in honor of Harold Hotelling* (pp. 278–292). Stanford University Press.

Ligges, U. (2009). *Programmieren mit R* (3rd ed.). Springer.

Loftus, G. R., & Masson, M. E. J. (1994). Using confidence intervals in within-subject designs. *Psychonomic Bulletin & Review, 1,* 476–490.

Lorch, R. F., & Myers, J. L. (1990). Regression analyses of repeated measures data in cognitive research. *Journal of Experimental Psychology: Learning, Memory, and Cognition, 16,* 149–157.

Mauchly, J. W. (1940). Significance test for sphericity of a normal n-variate distribution. *The Annals of Mathematical Statistics, 11,* 204–209.

Maxwell, S. E., Delaney, H. D., & Kelley, K. (2018). *Designing experiments and analyzing data: A model comparison perspective* (3rd ed.). Taylor & Francis.

McCormick, K., Salcedo, J., & Poh, A. (2015). *SPSS statistics for dummies*. John Wiley & Sons.

Mordkoff, J. T. (2019). A simple method for removing bias from a popular measure of standardized effect size: Adjusted partial eta squared. *Advances in Methods and Practices in Psychological Science, 2*, 228–232.

Morey, R. D., Rouder, J. N., Jamil, T., Urbanek, S., Forner, K., & Ly, A. (2019). BayesFactor (version 0.9.12-4.2) [Computer software]. https://cran.r-project.org/web/packages/BayesFactor/index.html

Neyman, J. (1967). *A selection of early statistical papers of J. Neyman*. Cambridge University Press.

Neyman, J., & Pearson, E. S. (1928). On the use and interpretation of certain test criteria for purposes of statistical inference. *Biometrika, 20A*, 175–240.

Nieuwenhuis, S., Forstmann, B. U., & Wagenmakers, E.-J. (2011). Erroneous analyses of interactions in neuroscience: A problem of significance. *Nature Neuroscience, 14*, 1105–1107.

Olejnik, S., & Algina, J. (2003). Generalized eta and omega squared statistics: Measures of effect size for some common research designs. *Psychological Methods, 8*, 434–447.

Pfister, R. (2021). Variability of Bayes Factor estimates in Bayesian analysis of variance. *The Quantitative Methods for Psychology, 17*, 40–45.

Pfister, R., & Janczyk, M. (2013). Confidence intervals for two sample means: Calculation, interpretation, and a few simple rules. *Advances in Cognitive Psychology, 9*, 74–80.

Pfister, R., & Janczyk, M. (2016). schoRsch: An R package for analyzing and reporting factorial experiments. *The Quantitative Methods for Psychology, 12*, 147–151.

Pfister, R., Schwarz, K. A., Carson, R., & Janczyk, M. (2013). Easy methods for extracting individual regression slopes: Comparing SPSS, R, and Excel. *Tutorials in Quantitative Methods for Psychology, 9*, 72–78.

Pierce, C., Block, R., & Aguinis, H. (2004). Cautionary note on reporting eta-squared values from multifactor ANOVA designs. *Educational and Psychological Measurement, 64*, 916–924.

Raftery, A. E. (1995). Bayesian model selection in social research. *Sociological Methodology, 25*, 111–164.

Rasch, B., Friese, M., Hofmann, W., & Naumann, E. (2010). *Quantitative Methoden. Einführung in die Statistik für Psychologen und Sozialwissenschaftler* (Vol. 1, 3rd ed.). Springer.

Rasch, D., & Guiard, V. (2004). The robustness of parametric statistical methods. *Psychology Science, 46*, 175–208.

Renkewitz, F., & Sedlmeier, P. (2007). *Forschungsmethoden und Statistik in der Psychologie*. Pearson.

Rosenbaum, D. A., & Janczyk, M. (2019). Who is or was E. R. F. W. Crossman, the champion of the Power Law of Learning and the developer of an influential model of aiming? *Psychonomic Bulletin & Review, 26*, 1449–1463.

Rosnow, R. L., & Rosenthal, R. (2003). Effect sizes for experimenting psychologists. *Canadian Journal of Experimental Psychology, 57*, 221–237.

Rouder, J. N., Speckman, P. L., Sun, D., Morey, R. D., & Iverson, G. (2009). Bayesian t tests for accepting and rejecting the null hypothesis. *Psychonomic Bulletin & Review, 16*, 225–237.

Scheffé, H. (1963). *The analysis of variance*. Wiley.

Schönbrodt, F. D., Wagenmakers, E. J., Zehetleitner, M., & Perugini, M. (2017). Sequential hypothesis testing with Bayes factors: Efficiently testing mean differences. *Psychological Methods, 22*, 322–339.

Shadish, W. R., Cook, T. D., & Campbell, D. T. (2002). *Experimental and quasi-experimental designs for generalized causal inference*. Houghton, Mifflin and Company.

Simmons, J., Nelson, L., & Simonsohn, U. (2011). False-positive psychology: Undisclosed flexibility in data collection and analysis allows presenting anything as significant. *Psychological Science, 22,* 1359–1366.

Simonsohn, U. (2013). Just post it: The lesson from two cases of fabricated data detected by statistics alone. *Psychological Science, 24,* 1359–1366.

Simonsohn, U., Nelson, L. D., & Simmons, J. P. (2014). P-Curve: A key to the file drawer. *Journal of Experimental Psychology: General, 143,* 534–547.

Spearman, C. (1910). Correlation calculated from faulty data. *British Journal of Psychology, 3,* 271–295.

Student. (1908). The probable error of a mean. *Biometrika, 6,* 1–25.

Tabachnick, B. G., & Fidell, L. S. (2012). *Using multivariate statistics* (6th ed.). Pearson.

Tendeiro, J. N., & Kiers, H. A. L. (2019). A review of issues about null hypothesis Bayesian testing. *Psychological Methods, 24,* 774–795.

Tschirk, W. (2014). *Statistik: Klassisch oder Bayes. Zwei Wege im Vergleich.* Springer Spektrum.

Ulrich, R., & Miller, J. (2018). Some properties of p-curves, with an application to gradual publication bias. *Psychological Methods, 23,* 546–560.

Wagenmakers, E.-J. (2007). A practical solution to the pervasive problems of p values. *Psychonomic Bulletin & Review, 14,* 779–804.

Wasserstein, R., & Lazar, N. (2016). The ASAs statement on p-values: Context, process, and purpose. *The American Statistician, 70,* 129–133.

Wasserstein, R., Schirm, A. L., & Lazar, N. A. (2019). Moving to a world beyond "$p < 0.05$". *The American Statistician, 73,* 1–19.

Welch, B. L. (1947). The generalization of 'Student's' problem when several different population variances are involved. *Biometrika, 34,* 28–35.

Wetzels, R., Matzke, D., Lee, M. D., Rouder, J., Iverson, G., & Wagenmakers, E.-J. (2011). Statistical evidence in experimental psychology: An empirical comparison using 855 t tests. *Perspectives on Psychological Science, 6,* 291–298.

Wilcox, R. R. (1987). New designs in analysis of variance. *Annual Review of Psychology, 32,* 29–60.

Wollschläger, D. (2010). *Grundlagen der Datenanalyse mit R. Eine anwendungsorientierte Einführung.* Springer.

Zar, J. H. (2005). Spearman rank correlation. In P. Armitage & T. Colton (Eds.), *Encyclopedia of biostatistics* (Vol. 7, 2nd ed.). John Wiley & Sons.

Index

© Springer-Verlag GmbH Germany, part of Springer Nature 2023
M. Janczyk, R. Pfister, *Understanding Inferential Statistics*,
https://doi.org/10.1007/978-3-662-66786-6

Printed in the United States
by Baker & Taylor Publisher Services